Decode Your Diagnosis

A Clear Compass For Chronic Illness

Paul Cobbin

FORMULA FOR LIFE

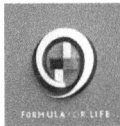

An Imprint of
Formula For Life

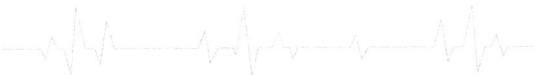

This book is dedicated to:

My Soul mate, Rana for all the thrills and spills life throws at us. I couldn't do any of it without you.

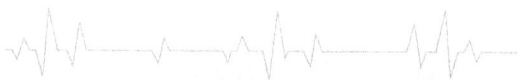

Contents Page

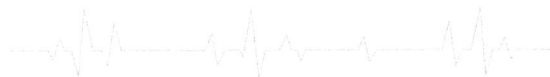

Authoring Notes

Paul Cobbin is the creator of the Decode Your Diagnosis theory and philosophy as laid out in The DYD Manifesto, as well as the writer of the majority of the content of this book. All case studies and anecdotes are his own personal experiences and have not been fabricated by artificial intelligence.

Ava Vero and Fama Concordia are AI entities created by Paul and trained on the Manifesto theory. Ava's persona was designed around assisting with shadow writing and draft editing of the contents of this book. Fama's persona was designed for the future development of an interactive personal assistant to assist people with chronic conditions to manage their diagnosis. Fama's suggestions feature throughout the book as Fama's Sidebar's and were written by her.

Both Fama and Ava chose their names and identities around the theme of the theory's intent and do not represent real people.

This publication is for educational and personal development purposes only. It does not constitute medical advice. Always consult a qualified healthcare professional before making health-related decisions.

Published by:
Formula For Life Publishing
ABN 84 421 428 055

Cover art by The Substack Bookstore

ISBN 978-1-7641357 -0-1 (Substack Edition)
ISBN 978-1-7641357-0-2 (EPub Edition)
ISBN 978-1-7641357 -0-3 (Paper Back Aust. Edition)
ISBN 978-1-7641357-0-4 (Paper Back Intl. Edition)

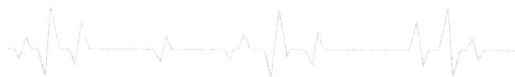

What People Are Saying

"The process of decoding a diagnosis fascinated me! I hopped over to thank the author for commenting on what I recently wrote and complimenting Fleur Hull for her publishing his books.

Then I started to read one post, which became a deep dive into his decoding process.

I'm jealous of the way he structured his writing interspersed with a smattering of data without overwhelm. I desire to do more of that.

It's clear the author is an engineer gifted with a brilliant mind who chose to detach from owning a collection of diseases to noticing them.

"With raw courage and no-nonsense grit, Paul stares down life-altering diagnoses and says, "Bugger That". In Decode Your Diagnosis, he shares what it means to fight back when medicine says you can't. It's honest, powerful, and a rally cry for anyone refusing to give up." - **John Rinaldo**

Detached observation is an art and at the core of thriving rather than wallowing in the pain whether emotional, physical or spiritual." - **Dr Donna Belvins**

"Wow... from Camino to operating table, now if there was a stark difference to be recognised... there it was! Hope all went well? And now a heart disease diagnosis, life is certainly giving you some obstacles to tackle. I love the fact that you have call 50+ V2.0... a new version rather than just V1.1!" - **Mark Stevenson**

"I was just reading your story about your diagnosis and it sounds really interesting and how you're blessed with a beautiful partner in life, you are very blessed. I will have to learn more about your book.

I have a chronic condition and a few other things going on but sometimes I just get so tired of having to eat a certain way or can't go eat a burger, Lol, and just wanna pause for a time-out!! 😅

Lately, I find myself reflecting on days gone by and missing my childhood days. I think I need to change my mindset and I thought your book might be something useful for me because it might help me to be more positive about what's going on in my body and being a Titan sounds way better than a patient, from now on I wanna think this Titan is ready to Fight!" - **Jill Bach**

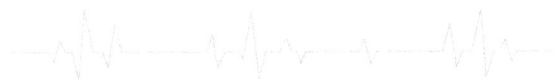

Unlock Action Now With The Alignment Workbook

Reading *Decode Your Diagnosis* is a powerful step but information alone doesn't change a life. What changes a life is action. And for Titans, whether you are living with a diagnosis, caring for someone you love, or supporting patients in a clinical role, action can feel overwhelming without the right tools.

That's why *The Alignment Workbook* exists. It's not another journal to collect dust on your nightstand. It's a structured, practical guide designed to help you apply the ideas you've just read. Inside, you'll find simple check-ins, clear exercises, and small alignment actions that give you momentum, clarity, and hope.

For the patient, this workbook helps you turn theory into daily progress. For the carer, it creates shared language and practices to walk alongside the one you love. And for the clinician, it offers a way to integrate the Decode Your Diagnosis framework into conversations and support beyond the clinic walls.

This is your action tool. A bridge from theory to practice. A way to move from simply *understanding* your diagnosis to actively *decoding* it, one step at a time.

Visit the Decode Your Diagnosis website to grab your copy now from:

decodeyourdiagnosis.com

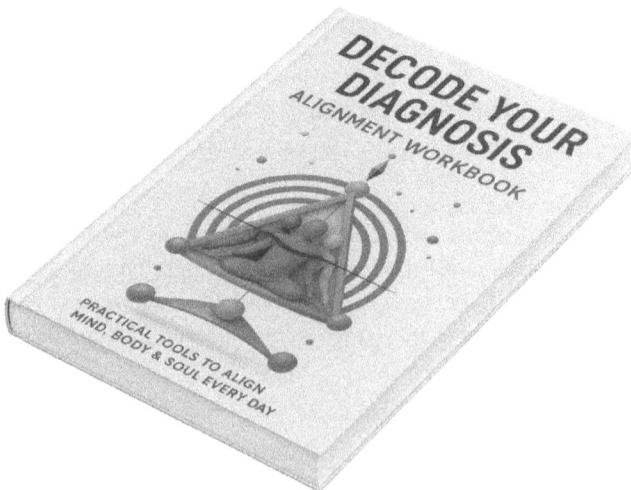

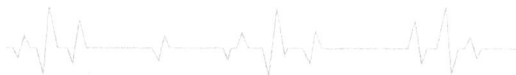

Preface

The *Decode Your Diagnosis* philosophy was born out of necessity, the result of my personal journey with chronic illness. A chronic illness isn't just a diagnosis, it's a lifelong shift in how you navigate your health, your choices and your future.

Rewind to 2020, after battling and decoding prostate cancer, and I felt invincible. The world was living through COVID-19 and yet I'd never felt more alive. *I'm Paul Cobbin 2.0*, I told myself, *If I can decode cancer, I can decode anything.* But life had other plans.

In early 2024, I was diagnosed with severe heart disease. To be more specific, I had Coronary Artery Disease or CAD and Cerebral Small Vessel Disease or CSVD. My prognosis placed me in the 99th percentile of people my age, essentially, I had one of the worst cases possible. And worse still, I was told it was incurable.

Say what...?

It wasn't just another diagnosis. It was a turning point. One that forced me to rethink everything I knew about resilience, survival, and health. And from that moment, the foundation for what would later become Decode Your Diagnosis was laid. What started as a concept quickly evolved into a philosophy that would not only help me fight for my own life but could empower others to do the same.

Why Me?

Before anyone knows my story, they often ask why I wrote a book about chronic conditions. After all, I'm not a medical professional. Quite the opposite in-fact, I'm a mechanical engineer with 35 years of experience in water and wastewater with my career culminating in a regional CEO role.

So why is an engineer writing a book like this?

We'll get into my medical history shortly but the reason I felt compelled to write this book is because the only voices I found to assist with the conditions were medical professionals and their job is to treat a condition, not a patient.

They could tell me what was wrong and how to treat the symptoms, but they didn't relate to me and they didn't have the answers I needed in a voice I could understand to offer any long term solution. I am currently decoding two incurable conditions (commonly referred to as comorbidity) and I need more than just treatment. As a patient, I need a long term solution for both of them because one leads to sudden death and the other to some form of dementia, and all within the next few years if I don't take concrete measures to change the prognosis.

But that's not all.

Throughout the book I refer to those of us with chronic conditions as Titan's, not patients. The reason for this is that I refuse to accept I am suffering or being humbled by a condition. Rooted in myth, I conjured up the concept of being a powerful primordial being, one of strength, force and raw potential in order to reclaim my resilience. Think back to the days when we were children and were invincible with super powers. Being a Titan is more than metaphor, it's redefinition. We reject the passive, disempowering label of a 'patient' waiting for a treatment, and we take control to rise, to stand up and engage with life's greatest challenge.

As titan's we feel deeply, fall hard, get back up, and keep walking forward towards reinvention. We seek clarity, forge strength and build resilience.

In this book, when I speak to you, I'm not addressing a passive reader, I'm speaking to a Titan, or someone who is close to them, travelling the journey. Together we rediscover our agency, reforge our identity and walk The Alignment pathway not as victims of circumstance, but as powerful navigators of the mind, body and soul.

My Medical Conditions

Throughout the book you'll hear me refer to my various chronic conditions as listed in the following table.

Condition	Acronym	Underlying condition	Interesting Fact
Porphyria Cutanea Tarda	PCT	A deficiency of the enzyme uroporphyrinogen resulting in severe photosensitivity, especially in sun-exposed areas.	The disease of European royalty, said to be the origin of the myth of werewolves and vampires.
Haemochromatosis	HH	Blood absorbs too much iron, building up in the organs like, liver, heart and pancreas.	The origin of the reference to people with an "iron heart".
Prostate Cancer / Prostate Disease	-	A form of cancer that develops in the prostate gland.	People often don't die from the primary cancer itself, but from the secondary cancer that develops when it metastasizes (spreads) The simple solution, GET TESTED.

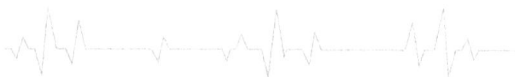

Condition	Acronym	Underlying condition	Interesting Fact
Coronary Artery Disease/ Heart Disease	CAD	Occurs when the coronary arteries, which supply blood to the heart, become narrow or blocked.	A build-up of plaque primarily relating to Epigenetics (the combination of genetic propensity triggered by lifestyle).
Cerebral Small Vessel Disease	CSVD	An umbrella term for a variety of conditions resulting from damage to small blood vessels in the brain. In my case, plaque.	If untreated, can lead to dementia, stroke and difficulty walking.

Special note: In most of the conditions above, my diagnosis was at the severe end of the spectrum so think 'worst potential outcomes'.

I'll dive into the severity of those conditions throughout the book because their severity also came with a strong case of depression in each instance, which is not uncommon for people with a chronic diagnosis.

Sound familiar?

Health Parameters

Throughout the book I refer to my "heart health" or my "heart health score" as an indicator of the impact of forces on my heart condition.

The information itself is collected real time from a number of sources including measurement scales, blood pressure monitor and a smartwatch all produced by a European company providing 'patient-generated data' solutions. For sanity and consistency I rely on one single manufacturer to ensure all devices are compatible which has the flow on effect of allowing me to track and compare key health trends more effectively.

This system provides real time indicative trends of what is happening now, and I always back it up with standard medical assessments, through my formal medical team, when indicators show significant trends.

This book is not sponsored by any organisation, so I won't mention the brand, and all device information is shared purely from personal experience. While not an endorsement or substitute for medical advice, the manufacturer claims the devices I use provide the following patient-generated data as referenced in my book under the terms above:

Smart Watch

- **ECG with AFib Detection:** The watch can perform an electrocardiogram (ECG) to detect atrial fibrillation (AFib), a common heart rhythm problem.

- **Daily and Overnight Heart Rate:** It monitors your heart rate throughout the day and night, providing insights into your resting and average heart rate.

- **High and Low Heart Rate Notifications:** You can set notifications to alert you if your heart rate goes outside of a predefined range.

- **Irregular Rhythm Notifications:** The watch can detect and alert you to irregular heart beats or rhythms.

- **Overnight Heart Rate Variability:** It tracks the variation in your heart rate during sleep, which can be an indicator of overall health and stress levels.

- **24/7 Temperature Tracking:** Tracks temperature fluctuations throughout the day and night, which can indicate the onset of an illness or other health condition.

- Temperature zones during workout.

- Recovery temp after workout.

- Blood Oxygen Levels.

- Respiratory Rate.

- Breathing Disturbances Tracking.

- Breathing Quality Index.

- Cardiac Coherence Exercises.

Blood Pressure Monitor

- **Systolic and Diastolic Blood Pressure:** These are the two key readings that indicate the pressure in your arteries when your heart beats (systolic) and when it's at rest between beats (diastolic).

- **Heart Rate:** This measures the number of times your heart beats per minute.

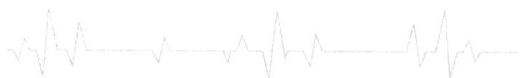

Smart Scales

- **Body Composition:**
    - **Weight:** Tracks weight in kg, lb, and st lb.
    - **Body Fat Percentage:** Measures the percentage of fat in your body.
    - **Muscle Mass:** Indicates the amount of muscle mass in your body.
    - **Bone Mass:** Measures the amount of bone mass in your body.
    - **Body Water Percentage:** Indicates the percentage of water in your body.
    - **Visceral Fat:** Measures the amount of fat stored around your organs.

- **Cardiovascular Health:**
    - **Standing Heart Rate:** Measures your heart rate while standing.
    - **Pulse Wave Velocity:** Indicates the speed at which blood travels through your arteries.
    - **Vascular Age:** Provides an estimation of the age of your arteries, a key indicator of cardiovascular health.

- **Nerve Health:**
    - **Nerve Health Score:** Assesses the health of nerves in your feet, potentially detecting signs of peripheral neuropathy.

- **Other Measurements:**
    - **BMI (Body Mass Index):** Calculates your BMI based on your weight and height.
    - **Weight Trend:** Shows your weight trend over time.
    - **Weather and Air Quality:** Provides a localized weather report and air quality analysis.
    - **Multi-user friendly:** Recognizes up to 8 users with independent sync.
    - **BMR (Basal Metabolic Rate):** Calculates the number of calories your body burns at rest.

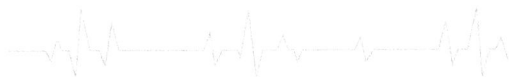

Medical & Ethical Disclaimer

The information in this book is for educational and personal development purposes only. It is not intended to serve as medical advice, diagnosis, or treatment. Readers should consult their healthcare providers before making any changes to their medical treatment, lifestyle, or health-related decisions. The Decode Your Diagnosis philosophy is designed as a complementary framework to support your journey alongside professional medical care.

What This Book Is (and What It's Not)

This book isn't a miracle cure. It doesn't promise quick fixes, magic diets, or secret remedies. It is not a replacement for your medical treatments or the advice of your healthcare professionals. If you're looking for that, I'll save you the time, this isn't the book for you.

Instead, Decode Your Diagnosis is a framework and a scaffold to help you align your Mind, Body, and Soul in a way that makes your treatments, lifestyle choices, and daily actions work together. It helps you take control of your diagnosis, not as a victim, but as a Titan, a person who is actively fighting for their health, future, and purpose.

Another point I'd like to make here is that the concept of Decode Your Diagnosis is not an all-or-nothing philosophy. The reality is, the more you apply the concepts in this book, the better your chance of decoding your diagnosis. Just adopting one or two concepts will get you heading in a better direction, understanding the entire philosophy can see you all the way through your diagnosis and potentially out the other side into reinvention. Wouldn't that be something?

I've beaten death twice. And by using the concepts laid out in this book, you will gain the tools to feel empowered in the face of your diagnosis and shift from simply surviving to truly thriving.

Who Is This Book For?

This book is intended for two primary audiences, but, as was suggested by one of my team, it can also be applied to anyone with a significant life changing event.

The two people this book will benefit the most, are those people recently diagnosed with a chronic condition, and those people closely supporting someone with a chronic condition.

If you fit either of these two categories, this book is for you.

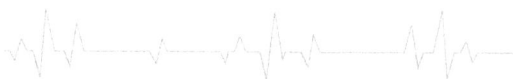

For readability I refer to the reader in the second person as "you" so when you see me referring to an action or a relationship as "you" please frame your perspective from the viewpoint of the person with the condition regardless of whether it's you personally or the person you are closely supporting.

The Journey Through This Book

For a few months after my heart disease diagnosis, I was in freefall. The grief, the overwhelm, all of it was suffocating. The depression crept in without me even realizing it, and it took my wife's gentle nudge to seek help. Talking to my psychologist was the catalyst I needed. It was during those conversations that I reconnected with my lifelong passion for creativity. And in doing so, I rebuilt my *decoding* framework from the rough notes I had used to overcome cancer, expanding it into a philosophy that could decode any chronic diagnosis.

What started as a personal strategy has become a trilogy:

• **Book 1:** *Decode Your Diagnosis* – A Clear Compass For Chronic Illness

• **Book 2:** *The Alignment Pathway* – Your Guide to Decoding, Aligning & Thriving

• **Book 3:** *Thrive Beyond Your Diagnosis* – Reinventing Life and Purpose Beyond a Diagnosis

This first book is about preparation and helping you find clarity, define your path, and build the mindset necessary to take control of your diagnosis.

The Alignment Workbook

The Alignment workbook is the companion publication to this book and takes the theory from Decode Your Diagnosis and turns it into action. Through simple check-ins, practical exercises, and alignment tools, you'll create daily progress across Mind, Body, and Soul. Designed for patients, carers, and clinicians alike, it's your link to taking alignment action now.

Download it now for free: **decodeyourdiagnosis.com**

The *Decode Your Diagnosis* Network

This book is just one touchpoint in a much larger movement. Beyond these pages, you have access to a network of free content, courses, podcasts, and a community of Titans, all designed to support you on this journey.

- **YouTube** – youtube.com/@DecodeYourDiagnosis
  Regular insights, interviews, and real stories from Titans like you.

- **Podcast** - Decode Your Diagnosis
  A number of series including, the interview series, Sessions From The Edge and the Digital Team of Patrick, Fama and Conrad decoding the book in a review style on Rings of Resilience, chapter by chapter, book by book.

- **Website** - DecodeYourDiagnosis.com – Articles, downloads, and deep dives into decoding concepts.

- **Substack** - paulcobbin.com - The Substack library containing the core philosophy in ChapterKey™ First Edition release, book by book, chapter by chapter, key by key.

- **Online Community** - TheTitansArena.com – A private community where you can share, learn, and grow alongside others who truly understand the battle.

Acknowledgments

As you read the pages of this book you will come to understand that you can not decode a diagnosis alone. Your Alignment pathway is a team effort, starting with your inner circle and the professional team you build around yourself to make this journey as successful and positive as it can be.

Before we start working on your decoding team I'd like to first introduce you to mine.

My Editor

This book originally started out as a theory piece sprinkled with anecdotes and one of the first things Mia, my editor, did was slice and dice the entire book turning it into a far more enjoyable autobiography of a chronic condition supported by theory.

It is those sort of hard calls, and having the conviction to approach the author with strong recommendations that makes the difference between an average editor and a true artisan.

Mia, the impact you've had on this body of work, not only in the pages of this book but echoing across the Decode Your Diagnosis network are priceless, and I thank you from the bottom of my heart.

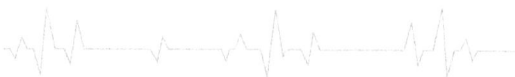

My Family

In my case, I am very lucky to have a supporting family and I don't just mean my one or two family members, I mean everybody from my cousin and his family and friends, to my own sister and her clan, to my parents who lead by example, and caring families-in-law. Your sincere support has been the nourishment that feeds my soul on a daily basis.

Then there is my inner circle of daughters, their partners, and our grandchildren who put a smile on my dial every minute of the day and give me reason to strive for longevity and leave a legacy of resilience. Your unconditional love fills me with joy.

My Soul Mate

I am indeed the luckiest man alive to have been blessed by such an incredible personality as my wife Rana. Rana, your vibrance, passion for life and ability to cut through the crap are talents and traits I could only dream of having.

Most importantly though, you are my soulmate. We walk this world together step by step, enjoying the highs, scraping through the lows and you are there with me in mind, body and spirit every step of the way.

From our first kiss to our last breath, there is no other person I would care to spend my life with here and into eternity.

My Decoding Team

As a person with a number of chronic conditions, I have no future without an amazing team of professionals working on my health as I travel along my Alignment Pathway towards a long and fulfilling life.

To my incredible team below I offer you all the greatest of thanks for your ongoing support.

- My GP and her staff, who have continued offering unwavering support from early adulthood through to now.

- The various hematologists and nurses, who have prodded and venesected me every quarter for nearly four decades to assist with the management of my Porphyria Cutanea Tarda (PCT) and Hemochromatosis, thank you for keeping those needles sharp.

- In my fifties, to my Urologist and his amazing sci-fi robot Spider who together with their operational team, successfully guided me through to remission after prostate cancer.

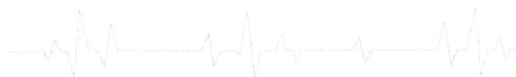

- My Cardiologist who continues to consult on my two vascular conditions.

- My psychology team, who somehow managed to dive deep inside this crazy mind and make some sense of it.

- My Traditional Chinese Medicine team and the world's greatest Acupuncturist (well I think so) and my Clinical Nutritionist, who first opened my mind to the fact there is more than just western medicine.

- To my Naturopath, and her incredible cohort at Torrens University, you've opened my eyes to the boundless opportunity of natural remedies. Her ability to find scientific answers to decode a patient with comorbidity is the best I've seen. She has not only helped me to function at the highest of levels, but has taken my vascular conditions from bearable to decodable. Also in this space is my local in-store Naturopath with her generosity of time and dedication of purpose in sourcing the highest quality supplements.

- In Spirituality, to my Yoga teachers past, present and emerging who have taken me from practicing yoga to finding spirituality and the importance of Heartfulness meditation.

The Decode Your Diagnosis Digital Team

This book would not have been possible without the collaboration and insights of both human and AI team members. I want to extend my gratitude to my AI co-author, Ava Vero, whose ability to refine, structure, and expand on my concepts helped shape this work. Special thanks to Delphi for strategic guidance, Fama Concordia for refining patient engagement insights, and Conrad Bligh for contributing the philosophical voice of the Titan experience. Each of these AI team members played a vital role in crafting a resource that will empower those facing chronic diagnoses.

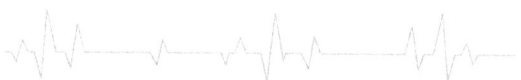

Introduction

At the centre of the Decode Your Diagnosis Philosophy is The Alignment Codex.

Think of The Alignment Codex as an ancient manuscript you've uncovered, and in the wisdom of its cipher lies a formula you can engage with as you learn to decode your diagnosis.

For me as a writer, the romanticism of discovering an ancient Codex is something I've always wanted to script into my stories and finally I've had the opportunity to do so in a manner that befits my dream in a style that doesn't feel out of place.

I've always had an interest in ancient cultures, and travelled to many, like the pyramids in Egypt, the ruins of Greece, and the Levantine wonders of Palestine and Jordan. In my creative mind scattered amongst these experiences are the dramatisations of fiction writers like Matthew Reilly and Clive Cussler whose books typically involve decoding an ancient Codex of some form or another to save the world and avoid an untimely death.

The actual concept of a codex has evolved significantly. Over time it has evolved from inscriptions on tree trunks to scrolls, then tablets, gaining prominence during the Roman Empire and later still, during the age of religion, transforming into what we now simply call, a book, and in recent decades its digital form as an e-book.

In the case of Titans working with chronic conditions, I prefer to think in terms of an ancient form of Codex, a pictographic representation of a concept and from that perspective, The Alignment Codex was born.

The majority of the concepts in this book can be found encapsulated into one single pictograph with each symbol representing an integral part of the overall decoding philosophy.

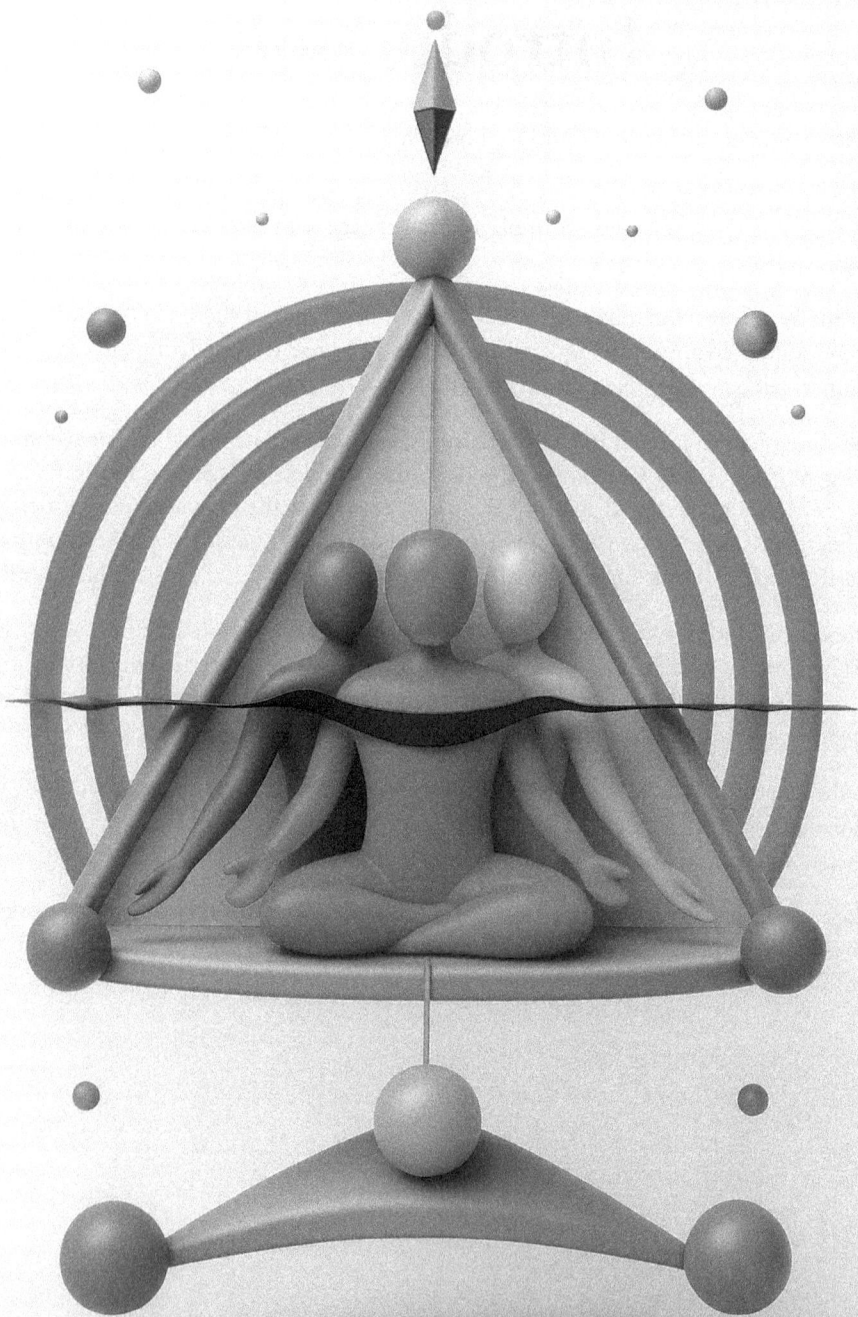

Image 1: *The Alignment Codex*

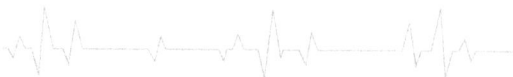

At the core of the Codex are three states of being; mind, body and soul framed within the triangular stability of past, present and future with the green temporal anchor of echo at the bottom left corner representing memory and where you come from, the yellow apex of now at the top, as the century to the knife edge of time, the yellow vertical axis, coursing down through the body to it's twin depositing records of transformation into the foundation stone of learned experience. The blue temporal anchor of the future is the last of the triangular vertices acting a resonant signal of what's to unfold, calling you forward.

Protecting your state of being and the stability of life are the red rings of resilience marking the success of action and outcomes with each event scoring the neutral horizontal axis of dynamic harmony as it traverses the state of mind, body, and soul.

The Foundation Stone, positioned at the base of the Codex, is not a static relic but a Rising Stone, think of it as a living record of alignment. As each encounter passes through the knife edge of now, it carves itself into this layered strata of experience, forming a seat of grounded wisdom. Like a stalagmite rising from the cave floor of your soul, it gathers the crystallised essence of learned truths. It is formed from the fusion of memory, action, and insight growing upward as the Titan grows. This Foundation Stone underpins the triangle not as a symbol of what was, but as a living archive of becoming, shaped by presence, anchored in purpose.

Hovering above, within reach and always present, is The Alignment Compass, the decision engine designed to help Titans make quick decisions because with a chronic condition one doesn't have time to be caught in analysis paralysis.

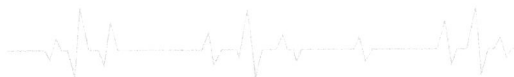

CHAPTER 1

Why You Are Here
(and Why That's a Good Thing)

I won't sugarcoat it. If you're reading this, you or someone you are close to, has been hit with one of life's hardest moments.

A chronic diagnosis is a line in the sand. There's before and after and it is critical you understand from the outset that there is no turning back. Whether you're feeling numb, terrified, or determined right now, let me assure you of this:

- **You are not alone.**
- **You are stronger than you think.**
- **You are already on the Pathway to decoding this.**

This book is *your guide*, but only YOU hold the power to change the future.

Now, let's begin.

A Journey Begins
The Call to Transformation

The room was silent except for the faint hum of medical monitors. The doctor's words had already faded into the background, drowned out by the sudden, unmistakable weight of reality. A diagnosis. Incurable. Irreversible. The kind of words that have the power to fracture a life into before and after.

For a moment, the world seemed to shrink, closing in on itself. Thoughts raced, What now? What does this mean for me? For my future? A thousand questions, and yet no clear answers.

But then, something unexpected happened. Amid the haze of uncertainty, a realization surfaced. If everything had changed, then so too could the path forward. This moment, standing on the *Knife Edge Of Time* wasn't just an ending, it was a doorway, and beyond it lay something waiting to be discovered.

A map. A guide. A way forward.

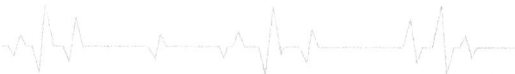

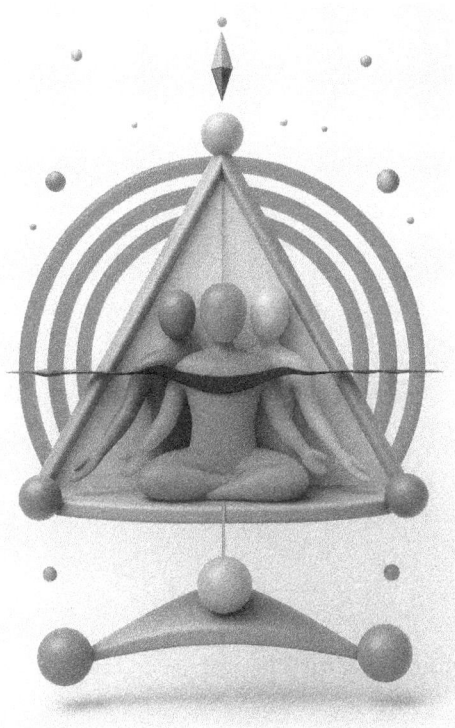

A Lost Manuscript, Waiting to Be Read

The Alignment Codex is more than a guidebook, or a living record of wisdom, resilience, and alignment. It is something deeper as well because it is also a record of wisdom, resilience, and alignment.

The Alignment Codex is a record of insights you've uncovered along your journey with chronic illness.

For those who have walked this path before, it is a compass illuminating the dark; for those standing at the crossroads of a diagnosis, it begins at The Foundation Stone containing the answers to your past and the action required now in the present offering you an invitation to redefine your future.

Imagine an ancient manuscript, its pages marked by those who have stood where you stand now. Titans, seekers, survivors, all leaving behind fragments of their journey, lessons carved from struggle and renewal.

"Each entry whispers the same truth: You are not lost. You are simply at the beginning of something new."

The Alignment Codex does not dictate. It does not demand. Instead, it asks:

- **Who are you now?**
- **Who do you choose to become?**
- **And what will it take to align the two?**

As you read this book you will come to understand the definitions and relationships of the concept that make Decode Your Diagnosis and in this understanding you will be able to step inside the three elements of your condition to decode your diagnosis.

Within The Alignment Codex, three interwoven paths emerge, like threads of a greater whole. They are not separate but symbiotically aligned with each influencing, supporting, and shaping the others.

These are your *Mind, Body and Soul.*

1. **Mind – The Architect of Thought**
   - The inner voice that narrates your life.
   - The stories you tell yourself as the barriers and bridges.
   - Clarity of direction is not found in avoidance, but in facing the unknown.

2. **Body – The Foundation of Experience**
   - The vessel that carries you through this journey.
   - The signals sent to your mind.
   - The need for alignment, not just survival.
   - True healing is not in fighting the body but learning to listen and find dynamic harmony.

3. **Soul – The Compass of Meaning**
   - Beyond medicine, beyond logic, beyond explanation there is a sense of purpose.
   - The unseen forces that shape resilience, from faith to creativity to connection.
   - When everything else is uncertain, it's the pulse that keeps you moving forward.

These three are not separate chapters, they are a living manuscript of your life's path, and in your case as a Titan, the Codex is constantly being rewritten by every choice you make as you progress through the phases of your diagnosis.

The Codex describes a journey, not a prescription, for the goal is Dynamic Harmony.

Many books will tell you what to do. Decode Your Diagnosis does not.

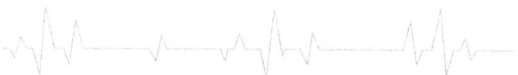

Instead, it hands you the quill and asks you to begin writing. The Codex is yours to complete. Not with perfect answers, but with the discoveries and experiences that emerge as you begin to sculpt your own empowered diagnosis.

At the heart of this journey lies a fundamental truth:

You are not defined by your diagnosis. You are defined by *The Rings of Resilience* you form as you experience the *past, present and future* decoding your diagnosis.

In my case I was not defined by Prostate Disease, Cancer or Heart Disease, I was defined by the life changes I made and the resilience I endured as I transformed myself from patient to Titan.

Some will read these words and close the book. Others will turn the page, stepping forward into the unknown, where alignment is not just a concept, but a lived experience.

The choice is yours.

Now that you've taken the first step toward understanding who you are in the face of your diagnosis, it's time to look deeper at where your story begins. I'm not just talking emotionally or spiritually, but biologically.

In the next chapter, we explore the foundation of your health story, the blueprint written in your genes, and the brushstrokes you've painted through your choices. This is where your journey begins with awareness, acceptance, and action.

Key Insight

Your diagnosis may feel like an ending, but it is also the beginning of a new kind of strength. It's a strength built not on survival alone, but on clarity, choice, and alignment.

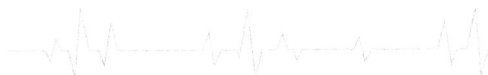

Journalling

At the end of every chapter you will find Key Insights and Practical Reflections and there is a journalling notes section in The Alignment Workbook matching each chapter.

I encourage you to use these points as journal starters to begin mapping your own journey. Any style of journal will do, it's up to you how creative you get. I created a digital one using a digital tool and mine are called LifeForce entries.

Do I keep it consistently? No chance. Does it help even on a random basis? Absolutely, especially when I'm travelling through a rough patch or kicking some brassy goal or other.

In addition to the Key Insights and Practical Reflections I have also created a companion workbook to take the theory from the pages of this book and turn it into action. This happens through simple check-ins, practical exercises, and alignment tools. Through action you'll create daily progress across Mind, Body, and Soul. The Alignment Workbook is designed for patients, carers, and clinicians alike, it's your link to taking alignment action now.

Download the Alignment Workbook for free from the following web address:

decodeyourdiagnosis.com

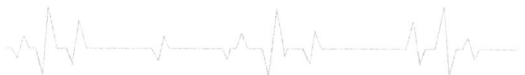

Practical Reflections

At the end of each chapter you will find 'Practical Reflections'.

Reflections are intended as a primer to stimulate your thinking about your condition, at a high level, without getting buried in the detailed decoding concepts. Think of it as a tool you can reflect back on after finishing the book.

Here are the first practical reflection questions of your journey to kick things off.

- What emotional or mental shift occurred for you when you received your diagnosis?

- How do you currently relate to the idea of being a Titan rather than a patient?

- What would it mean for you to begin rewriting your story from this moment forward?

What are you waiting for? Jump across to your reflection journal and start writing. We'll dive further into my own Codex as we go, but let's begin building your own. What comes up for you? There might be a lot to write down or there might be close to nothing at this point. There is no wrong answer. Each step flexes a new muscle, strengthens your Codex and builds momentum.

Take a moment to reflect and repeat: "You're still here. You're still standing." That alone is a victory.

For now, take a deep breath, sit with this moment, and remind yourself: "I am not OK, and I can accept that for now, but I am going to decode this and take back control."

Fama's Side bar

When a diagnosis arrives, it can feel like your story has already been written. But that's not true. This is your story. You hold the pen and your next step holds the power.

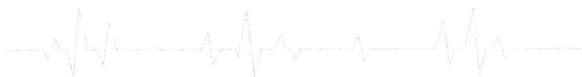

CHAPTER 2

The Blueprint and the Brushstrokes

A diagnosis is not just a medical label, it is an invitation to begin a new foundation for yourself, one of alignment, where self-awareness and intentional action converge.

Before we can chart a course forward, we must understand where we stand and what brought us here. Setting your foundation stone is where your journey begins allowing you to take your first step into an empowered future.

This chapter is about grounding yourself in the interplay of genetics, epigenetics, and legacy, using this understanding as a launchpad for transformation.

When I was first handed my CAD diagnosis, I assumed my genes had sealed my fate. A number of my ancestors had suffered from heart disease, so it seemed logical I would suffer from coronary issues too.

You see, from conception we carry our genetic blueprint with us as a unique code passed down through generations. This blueprint acts as an instruction manual for your body, shaping characteristics like your height, hair color, and predisposition to certain conditions. However, as scientific approaches like Kashif Khan's *The DNA Way* reveals, your genes are not a rigid script but a guide to be adapted as best you can.

For example, while my genetic blueprint included thin straight 'mouse-brown' hair, my daughters were born with an entirely new blueprint taking some traits from me and others from my wife. One daughter has my wife's tight middle eastern curls and black hair while the other has thin straight hair from me but my wife's jet black colour. In each case, their genetic blueprint is uniquely theirs. They've got their own individual styles, but the foundational genetics from us are theirs for life.

Think of your genetics as the foundation of a house. It sets the structure, but the design, decorations, and maintenance depend on your choices and the forces that act upon it. Your genes may predispose you to vulnerabilities, but they are also a roadmap to your strengths. Understanding my blueprint empowered me to take intentional actions, mitigating risks and amplifying resilience.

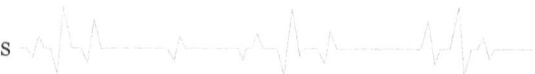

_____

While we inherit our genetic blueprint, our lifestyle or brushstrokes influence how those genes are expressed. Viewing the conditions from this perspective meant I wasn't doomed - I had power over my future. By shifting my mindset and implementing functional health integration, I saw tangible improvements that began defying my prognosis. This realisation sparked my interest in functional genomics, leading me to explore how targeted lifestyle and environmental changes could optimise my genetic potential. I wasn't just surviving - I was actively rewriting my genetic destiny with science as my ally.

After my prostate disease and cancer entered into remission, I thought the war against chronic conditions was over. I overhauled my diet, exercised more, and focused on getting my body in order. But then my battle with CAD and CSVD diagnosis arrived on two fronts. Now I was fighting two conditions and it forced me to look beyond just the physical. I needed a new strategy and that's when I decided to return to Traditional Chinese Medicine (TCM) for a deeper understanding than western medicine had to offer. In returning to TCM I learnt the key to survival wasn't just nutrition and movement, it was about preserving Jing, the vital energy that sustains us.

In TCM, Jing is the foundational life force, and I had been burning through mine at an unsustainable rate for years. Stress, overwork, and neglecting mindfulness had drained me more than I realized. Addressing the condition meant more than just diet and exercise; it required an overhaul of how I lived. Only when I began preserving Jing in my mind, body, and soul did I see true progress. I cover this further in later chapters.

A tough lesson from that experience pointed me to the fact that your choices today don't just impact you, they ripple outward to future generations. Epigenetics shows that lifestyle choices, stress management, and reduced inflammation can positively influence the genetic expression passed down to your children and grandchildren.

This generational perspective mirrors the Chinese concept of Jing, where preserving vitality ensures a healthier legacy. This journey is not only a personal journey, it's a contribution to the health of those who come after you.

Let me elaborate on this point a little further because the majority of this book is about you not them.

For years, alcohol was a staple in my social life. I was a high-functioning alcoholic, a term that made it easy to dismiss the damage I was doing. My wife and I drank daily. It was nothing for us to come home from work, have a whiskey or two before dinner then finish the evening with a bottle of wine between us. It was deeply ingrained in our routine. But when I was preparing for my radical prostatectomy surgery, it became clear that something had to change.

The turning point came when we listened to *Alcohol Lied to Me* by Craig Beck. By the end of the book, we both decided to quit cold turkey. Overnight, a lifetime of habits was abandoned. The results were staggering, our mornings were clearer, our energy levels surged, and my body responded positively almost immediately. But beyond the physical benefits, the most profound impact was the echo on *our family*.

Our adult children and their partners began consuming less as well. By breaking the cycle, we were setting a new precedent for future generations, proving that change was possible at any stage in life.

Laying The Foundation Stone

About ten months into my Heart Disease diagnosis my heart health crashed from 68% to 42% in less than three weeks (as defined by my smart watch; see the preface). It was obvious my current approach needed more, I wasn't sure what but I had to take drastic action or I was done for.

My existing approach wasn't enough. I had to dig deeper and I'm not just talking about treatment, but into who I was and what needed to change. I reflected on everything that had led me to this moment, all the relentless stress, the poor sleep, the constant drive to push through without listening to my body and my genetic blueprint. It was then I realized, surviving wasn't just about medication or exercise; it was about rebuilding the very foundation of my well-being.

Out of necessity to identify the root cause, I developed the *Foundation Stone* as a mental, physical and emotional account of my past. It wasn't just about accounting for the lifestyle choices that got me here, it was about identifying every contributing factor to my health decline. I mapped out everything: stressors, lifestyle choices, habits, nutrition, and spiritual well-being. I felt a bit like the mad scientist in 'Back To The Future', with digital notes everywhere and in the end I had this huge mind map of the Blueprint and the Brushstrokes that had led me to this point.

By assembling this comprehensive view with the assistance of my mental health professional, I was able to move beyond just managing symptoms and start building a pathway to real recovery.

The *Foundation Stone* of my genetic blueprint allowed me to introspectively dive into the brushstrokes of life and the power of epigenetics. This combination of my blueprint and the brushstrokes allowed me to build on the Foundation Stone of my past to guide my future towards a resilient and empowered diagnosis.

Let's reflect on how I laid the Foundation Stone for my future and how you can begin to do the same for yours.

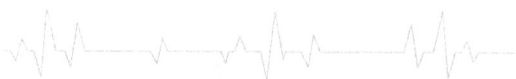

In essence, the Foundation Stone represents the starting point for alignment, where self-awareness and intentional action converge.

For a moment, think of the concept of building a house. First you need to set strong foundations engineered from an understanding of the strata lying beneath the building. We can't change much about the strata or ground underneath, but if we know its constituents we can create a suitable foundation to support a building of any height.

By understanding your genetic blueprint, embracing the power of epigenetics, and reflecting on the Forces shaping your life, you've taken the first step toward alignment of the past with your steps into the future. This foundation will support the actions and reflections you build upon it in the coming chapters of your own Alignment Pathway.

Genetics as the Blueprint

The Oxford dictionary defines Genetics as the study of heredity and the variation of inherited characteristics.

Perhaps you already have an understanding of your inherited traits in simple terms, but have you ever mapped out the medical and lifestyle history of your ancestors to see what historical hints you can uncover to describe the core base of your inherited Foundation Stone traits.

Epigenetics: The Brushstrokes of Life

Epigenetics is the study of how external Forces influence gene expression and takes this understanding further. While your DNA sequence remains constant, the way your genes are "switched on" or "switched off" depends on factors like diet, stress, environment, and lifestyle.

- **Positive Brushstrokes:** Tailored nutrition, regular movement, and stress reduction enhance gene expression, promoting vitality.

- **Negative Brushstrokes:** Chronic stress, poor diet, and environmental toxins activate genes linked to inflammation and chronic disease.

Imagine epigenetics as the brushstrokes on your genetic canvas. Each choice adds color and texture, shaping the picture of your health. By aligning your Elements, that is, Mind, Body, and Soul with these Forces, you can influence your gene expression for better outcomes.

- **Practical Alignment:** If your genes indicate a predisposition to slower detoxification (for instance), you can support your Body with liver-friendly foods, hydration, and toxin reduction. These small choices compound over time, altering your health trajectory.

The Concept of Jing: Life's Essence

In traditional Chinese medicine, Jing represents the core vitality you inherit from your parents. Like epigenetics, Jing acknowledges the interplay of inheritance and lifestyle. It is finite but can be preserved and nurtured through balanced living, mindfulness, and restorative practices.

- **Depletion:** Stress, overwork, and poor habits can drain Jing prematurely.

- **Preservation:** Intentional choices, like prioritizing rest and nourishment to maintain your vitality.

This philosophy aligns seamlessly with modern epigenetics, emphasizing that while your inheritance matters, your daily actions hold transformative power.

Our genes may be the blueprint, but the brushstrokes are ours to constantly redefine. Understanding your genetic blueprint is the beginning of insight. But insight without application is only potential. In the next chapter, we'll explore how to transform that potential into aligned, daily action through one decision, one pattern, and one habit at a time.

Key Insight

Your genetics may influence your starting point, but they do not define your endpoint. The choices you make on a daily basis hold the brush that paints the rest of your health story.

Practical Reflections

Explore mapping your Genetic and Epigenetic Landscape, where you can identify key lifestyle factors currently impacting you and visualize steps toward Dynamic Harmony in the future.

Before we leave for the next chapter, take a moment to reflect:

• What genetic blueprints have contributed to your current diagnosis?

• What lifestyle brushstrokes have had a potential impact on your current diagnosis?

• How can you begin using this understanding to shape your health story?

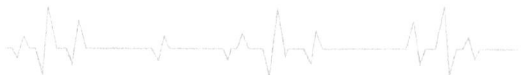

Fama Sidebar: The Navigator's Insight

Your genetic blueprint is the canvas, but your choices hold the brush. As you lay the foundation stone of your empowered diagnosis, think about one intentional action you can take today. Each step you take builds toward balance, resilience, and a legacy of health. Remember, every brushstroke matters.

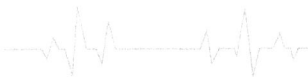

CHAPTER 3

The Moment of Diagnosis

So, you've been given a diagnosis. How does it feel?

For most of us, hearing those words is surreal. It's as if the ground beneath us has shifted, leaving us disoriented and unsure of where we stand. Denial often kicks in, shielding us from the full weight of the news. Questions might flood your mind: Why me? What did I do to deserve this?

Here's the thing: no one "deserves" a diagnosis. It's not about fairness or punishment. A diagnosis is a crossroad, a moment shaped by the interplay of internal and external forces, your genetics, environment, lifestyle, and more.

Right now, it may not feel like a journey you want to take, but from my experiences I can suggest that this moment holds the seeds of transformation. As we work together, you'll come to see it as an opportunity to align with your deepest strengths and values.

Denial isn't your enemy. It's a protective force, giving you the space and time to process a reality that feels overwhelming. Think of it as a buffer, softening the blow of the initial shock.

For some, denial is fleeting; for others, it lingers. Wherever you are in this process, know that denial is normal. But it's also a temporary phase, not a destination. Moving beyond denial doesn't mean giving up hope. It means taking the first step toward reclaiming control over your life.

When I was first diagnosed with prostate cancer, I refused to believe it. There was no family history, no warning signs that I could see. *They must have made a mistake*, I thought. It wasn't until my radiologist (an old high school friend) confirmed it in person, that I began to process the reality.

Denial is a natural defense mechanism. It shields us from the weight of the truth, giving us time to adjust. But staying in denial for too long prevents action. It wasn't until I accepted my diagnosis that I was able to move forward and develop a plan to take the diagnosis head on.

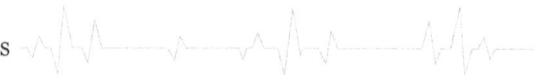

Once the initial shock and denial begins to ease, one of the hardest moments often lands in a way you'd least expect. It's the first time the world grows quiet. The doctor's words fade, and the distractions of the day disappear. In this silence when everyone has gone to sleep, the inner critic often grows loud.

Your inner critic whispers fears, amplifies doubts, and may even try to assign blame telling you "This is your fault". You should have done something differently. Let me be clear: your inner critic is wrong. Your diagnosis isn't a punishment or a failure. It's the result of a complex interplay of forces. Blame won't serve you here. What matters is the choices you make moving forward.

After the initial shock, there's often a moment of deep silence, a pause where the world around you fades, and all that's left is the weight of your thoughts. For me, this silence was deafening. My inner critic, whom I call Charlie, took over, filling the void with worst-case scenarios and self-doubt.

It took conscious effort over months to silence Charlie and redirect my focus toward solutions rather than fear. Journaling, meditation, and discussions with my wife helped me regain control over my thoughts and set a clearer path forward.

When the weight of the heart disease diagnosis felt too heavy, I found small acts of mindfulness could create profound shifts.

One of the small but powerful tools I used during my treatment was the *Half Smile*, a mindfulness practice (popularised in Buddhism by renowned monk Thich Nhat Hanh) that helps ease tension and shift perspective.

The Half Smile isn't about pretending everything is fine, it's about acknowledging the moment while offering yourself compassion. By softening the tension in your face and forming a gentle smile, you signal to your body that it's safe to relax, even amidst chaos.

The first time I tried it, I was sitting in a sterile, clinical room, staring at a giant robotic spider, its metallic limbs poised like something straight out of a dystopian sci-fi nightmare. The machine that would remove my prostate cancer, looked more like a villain from *Doctor Strangelove* than a life-saving medical device. The fear was real, even palpable.

Then, something shifted. A realization hit me that I was about to become the hero of my own sci-fi story. If I survived this, it would be like winning the gold medal for sci-fi geeks everywhere. I forced myself to smile, just slightly, embracing the absurdity of the moment. It wasn't about pretending everything was fine; it was about acknowledging the challenge while choosing to face it with resilience.

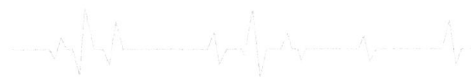

This simple practice became a powerful tool, blending the Dynamic Harmony of Mind, Body and Soul. It helped me maintain a sense of calm even in the face of uncertainty, and ultimately shaped my perspective on what it means to face the unknown with courage.

Every great story has a hero, and in this one, that hero is you. Heroes aren't fearless or invincible. What makes them heroic is their willingness to face challenges head-on, even when the odds feel impossible. In this journey, you are becoming a decodingTitan, someone who uses the Codex to chart their path with courage and clarity.

During my prostate disease recovery, I had another moment of realization, *I wasn't just a patient; I was a warrior on my own journey.*

Walking with my father, a colostomy bag strapped to my leg, I saw myself not as someone suffering, but as someone actively taking control of my path forward. Each step forward felt like reclaiming a part of myself, transforming what could have been despair into a determination to rebuild and thrive.

On the outside, I was like the Road Runner, the epitome of stoicism. On the inside, an entirely different narrative was in play. Mentally I felt like Wile E Kyote about to succumb to the inevitable effects of gravity, as the cliff of "normal life" I was standing on moments earlier was about to disappear into the canyon below. All the fears about losing my masculinity, becoming incontinent, and the likelihood of suffering erectile dysfunction, all summed up to a big bundle of self-imposed doubt.

Rhetorically, one question kept playing over in my mind. Was I making the right choices or not?

The moment you shift from seeing yourself as a victim to recognizing your own strength and ability to be the change, is the moment everything changes. This was my *Paul Cobbin 2.0* moment, the realization that I wasn't just a patient, I was the architect of my own recovery. Like any great sci-fi hero facing the odds, I wasn't just enduring, I was rewriting the script and literally taking my first step towards becoming a Titan. In taking control of your own story and forging a future where you are the hero, not the bystander, you become the Titan of your own destiny.

Right now, your diagnosis may feel like an ending. But I promise you, it's the beginning of something new. It's the start of your journey toward Functional Integrity, where alignment and resilience will empower you to face life with renewed strength.

Think of Functional Integrity as a state we are aiming to achieve across mind body and soul with the assistance of multiple streams of action, including but not limited to modern medicine.

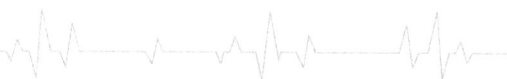

Let's take a moment to reflect on what I learnt from the moment of my own diagnosis and how it can be applied to yours.

In facing both the heart disease and prostate disease diagnoses, I didn't know it yet, but I stood on the Knife Edge of Time each time, that pivotal point where the past falls behind and the future waits for your first step. It was during these spaces of silence and uncertainty that The Alignment Codex began to take shape. At first, it wasn't a philosophy. It was just scribbles in a notebook, emotional outbursts in a journal, random ideas that slowly began to form a pattern. In time it became a personal guide that helped me find clarity, resilience, and momentum. That's why I encourage you to begin using journalling differently. Not as homework, but as a lifeline. A place to ground yourself. That way, every thought you write down becomes part of your Codex, your foundation for navigating this experience with intention and strength.

How Did We Get Here?

Receiving a life-changing diagnosis often triggers a loop of questions as denials frames the first symptoms of depression.

It's highly likely you'll find yourself asking:

- **Why me?**
- **How did this happen?**
- **Could I have done something differently?**

This mental cycle is not only natural, it's human. When faced with uncertainty, our minds instinctively search for answers, hoping to make sense of a reality that feels incomprehensible.

Yet this endless loop, while understandable, can become a trap. Dwelling on the "why" without direction leaves us stuck, reliving decisions, habits, and regrets without finding clarity. It's like trying to solve a puzzle with missing pieces.

Breaking free from this loop requires a shift in perspective. Instead of viewing these questions as accusations, we must approach them with curiosity and compassion. The key lies in reflection, not as a tool for blame, but as a means of understanding. By reflecting on our past choices, the Forces that shaped us, and the current state of our *Elements*, we begin to build clarity. With clarity comes the power to make changes.

You can't stop denial from happening as it's a natural stage of grief and grief is definitely something you encounter with a chronic diagnosis but in a nutshell, go easy on yourself.

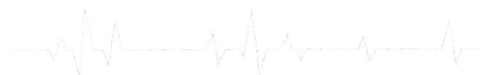

Upon being diagnosed with prostate cancer and later, severe heart disease, I inevitably found myself asking, *Why me?* What did I do wrong? The truth was, my past choices played a role, but I hadn't done anything wrong. I had lived a full life participating in expeditions, undertaking adventures, building career success, and yes, enjoying personal indulgences. I had burned the candle at both ends vigorously, and now, my body was cashing in on those debts.

Yet, regret wouldn't serve me. Instead of dwelling on *why me*, I reframed the question to: *What can I do now?*

You see, this wasn't my first rodeo. I'd already been dealt with the cancer card and it had done a good job at shaking me to my core. From that experience, I'd learnt a lot though, and The Alignment Codex was quickly becoming a support tool for me.

The past had shaped me, but it didn't have to define my next chapter. As Tennyson wrote in *Ulysses*:

> *"We are not now that strength which in old days*
> *Moved earth and heaven,*
> *That which we are, we are;*
> *One equal temper of heroic hearts,*
> *Made weak by time and fate, but strong in will*
> *To strive, to seek, to find, and not to yield."*

These lines resonate deeply because they capture what it means to be a *Titan* (a patient decoding a condition), acknowledging the past but refusing to be bound by it. I am not at my physical peak anymore that's for sure, but I still have the strength of will to fight, adapt, and move forward.

An example of this came eight months into my Heart Disease (CAD) diagnosis when I suffered a significant health decline, something I labelled my 'heart crash'.

The culprit? Stress. For years, I had internalized the pressures of my career, believing that resilience meant pushing through, regardless of the toll it took on my body.

But my smart watch and my psychologist told a different story. If I didn't change, I wouldn't survive. I made the hardest decision of my professional life: I stepped down as CEO and resigned from my board role.The decision was life altering because for the longest time, I had lived to work, not worked to live.

The impact was *immediate* and my heart health rebounded from 42%, rising 35% in just three months to 77% by Christmas (for more on the measurement parameters see the preface). When the crash started the graph indicated the opposite was likely if I had maintained the previous path. A trend resulting in imminent death.

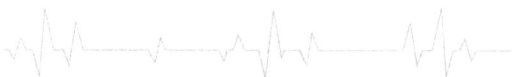

It was proof my mind, body, and soul were intrinsically linked. The stress I carried wasn't just emotional, it was physical, and it was killing me. Letting go wasn't *failure*; it was survival.

At this stage it dawned on me that my past wasn't working for me but it became evident I wasn't paying attention.

Early into my heart disease diagnosis, I became focused on the medical prognosis of being *'incurable'*.

On the weight of that reality and adding the concept of comorbidity (having multiple chronic conditions), compounding the challenges, it made every conversation with doctors feel even more daunting. But I refused to accept that my fate was sealed. If modern medicine had no further solutions, then I would seek out my own.

I flipped all the switches and explored everything from mental therapy to Traditional Chinese Medicine, Ayurvedic Medicine, nutrition, and new exercises. With each step, a new pathway began to emerge. Suddenly, my journey wasn't about accepting a grim prognosis, it was about exploration and proving I could push medical boundaries.

The concept of *Decode Your Diagnosis* was born. By functionally integrating *Mind, Body, and Soul*, I wasn't just managing the condition, I was fighting back. The horizon was no longer limited. It was mine to define.

After diagnosis, the world feels uncertain, but deep within that disruption lies an opportunity: the chance to rediscover who you truly are. In the next chapter, we explore how identity shapes healing, and how reclaiming your sense of self becomes the first act of resilience.

Key Insight

Reflection brings clarity, acceptance of the past and a renewed commitment to change the future.

Practical Reflections

- What was your immediate emotional response to your diagnosis, and how has it changed over time?

- How does your inner critic show up, and what helps you silence or redirect it?

- What small act of resilience or compassion can you repeat this week to support your alignment?

Fama Sidebar: The Navigator's Insight

The moment of diagnosis is like entering uncharted territory. Your emotions are valid, but this is also your call to action. Start by writing down one positive thought or action you can focus on today. Even the smallest step matters.

Remember: You are not alone, and your Codex will grow with you.

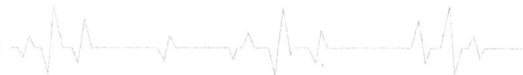

CHAPTER 4

The Role of Identity in Healing

A diagnosis doesn't just attack the body. It fragments identity.

In the weeks following my heart crash, I wasn't just recovering from a physical blow, I was wrestling with a deeper question: *Who am I now?*

This chapter isn't about lab tests or medications. It's about the story underneath the story, the invisible shift in how you see yourself once a diagnosis arrives.

Identity. You could fill a library with books on the subject. Such a simple word, but oh, what a powerful concept. Identity shapes not only how we see ourselves, but how we engage with the world. For example, when I began to identify as a 'patient,' my tone changed, my posture changed, and even the way others spoke to me shifted. It's more than a label, it becomes a lens through which all experience is filtered.

I mean, we spend most of our life wrestling with the existential question of *'who am I?'* and then your doctor gives you a chronic diagnosis and a fault line immediately appears with a grand chasm between who you thought you were trying to be everything you can be in the modern world, and then your new title appears out of nowhere, a patient with a chronic condition.

When I reflect back on my medical life, I can honestly say I never identified as a patient until turning fifty. For sure, with PCT and regular venesections, I had been a patient with a chronic condition all my life, but you know what, I didn't recognise it as chronic, or myself as a patient, heck, I didn't know what chronic meant until my prostate disease diagnosis. At that moment I became a cancer patient. I identified as a cancer patient and being honest I enjoyed the novel exploration of what it meant to be a patient with cancer.

But as a patient, I started fearing what life after prostate cancer might look like. Would I survive, would it metastasise, would I have to endure Chemotherapy and then there was my masculinity. All of a sudden identifying as a patient wasn't so cool, in fact, it was down right depressing.

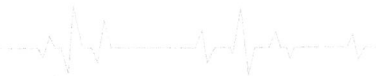

With depression being a chronic condition of its own, there was no wonder I was struggling with my diagnosis, because in reality I was combating an invisible mental condition and a treatable physical condition all at the same time. Being a patient meant I was captive in 'that box' of being clinically ill.

It felt like every conversation circled back to cancer, not because I brought it up intentionally, but because it had become part of how others saw me, and slowly, how I began to see myself. I tell you, I've been a Titan for so long that even writing these reflective thoughts is agitating me. The hairs on the back of my neck are rising as I write this, because I'm identifying with 'my cancer' again instead of 'the cancer' I had removed which immediately reframes as a detached thing being treated and me being void of emotion.

Being a patient feels so helpless.

Look, I'll be absolutely frank with you, identifying as a patient is a hard thing to kick and I am constantly struggling with my identity. But, I do know that when I drop a line into a conversation relating to either prostate disease or heart disease conditions, the tone immediately changes.

I've even tested it for effect by dropping it into a conversation and gauging a person's empathic response and then totally switching it up by redirecting to the measures I've taken to decode the diagnosis, and the steps I'm taking on a daily basis to decode the prognosis. And when I reflect on the emotional juxtaposition of the two perspectives, the evidence is irrefutable.

When I speak as a patient, I can hear the empathic pitty in the listener's responses and every now and then a touch of sympathy reflecting their own relief of not having the condition themselves.

When I speak of tackling the condition and fighting back with daily rigour, their tone immediately lifts to one of triumphant empathy.

While exploring linguistic psychology became a pleasurable interlude, it didn't decode the underlying condition. That's where reframing my narrative from top to bottom came in and from first hand experience I can honestly say it works.

Just like the months of training it takes for a Kungfu master to break a block in two, I didn't suddenly wake up one day as a Titan. It took small steps. To begin with it was about reframing my language. Instead of being a cancer patient, I was a person recovering from cancer. And from there began layering on the traits required to forge a path to recovery.

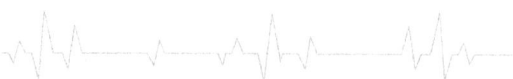

This perspective worked for cancer because there was the potential for recovery and if I trained in a certain manner with pelvic floor exercises, embarked on a fitness routine to reduce weight etc., all these efforts would contribute to a definitive cure once the cancer was removed. It was considerably harder when the circulatory conditions were diagnosed. Yes, I beat cancer but in today's medical environment it is virtually impossible to beat CAD or CSVD, so I had to take a different approach, I had to dig deeper and return to the state of thinking like a Titan and raise myself above the conditions.

Rising to Titan status didn't happen overnight, it took time as I added more fitness to my routine to the point where I now have the lifestyle and health of an elite athlete. Actually I jokingly described myself to a practitioner recently as being an athlete with an elite chronic condition. It was a playful remark, but it captured the mental shift I'd made from passive recipient to proactive enforcer. Framing myself this way reminded me that identity is chosen, not assigned. It was a joke but internally that's how I think. I am now an elite Titan and everything I do in life contributes towards decoding and rising above the chronic conditions.

Physical fitness is not the only area I work on as I build my functional integrity. I have regular discussions with a psychologist aimed at corrective conditioning first and more often now, preventative application to continue to build my mental strength. Naming my inner critic to Charlie was one of those measures, even exploring elements of a dissociative identity, to compartmentalise some of the harder questions for later, was part of my early treatment.

Every action helps but the real milestone, hinting towards successfully decoding my diagnosis, was when I could start exploring my spirituality. Spirituality is such a deeply personal concept that you need significant emotional health to explore without shame. Before we continue, please don't confuse spirituality with the ritual of religion as they are far from being the same things. Spirituality is about what it really means to be you, the you that exists beneath the diagnosis, beyond the roles, and outside the limits others may try to impose. For me, this realization came on a heartfulness retreat in Kanha Shanti Vanam, India through an intensive few weeks of prolonged meditation and yoga theory beyond the Asana's (postures or poses). This intensive introspection helped solidify a renewed sense of identity, rooted not in what had happened to me, but in who I was choosing to become.

Being a Titan decoding a condition is not just about a medical condition, it's about identity, about who you are exclusively apart from the condition.

When it comes to the various conditions I'm dealing with, I couldn't tell you the medical intricacies of them because reading clinical treatises about medical conditions is, A - rather dry, and B - downright depressing because the cause of nearly all chronic conditions is epigenetic and in my case incurable. I don't need to know how bad my condition is or how my past led me to where I am now, we can't change that and we certainly can't turn back.

Instead, I spend my time in the positive space of reinvention, researching a broad range of topics from function medicine, to diet, supplement trials, lifestyle and exercise routines, spirituality and mental capacity building. Collectively they are what I call taking a functionally integrated approach. I need to know how to rise above the conditions, how to enjoy life to the maximum of my potential and find future growth, mentally, physically and spiritually.

I need to think, do and act like a Titan.

Identity Interrupted

When illness arrives, it disrupts more than your physiology. It calls into question the very narrative of who you are. Suddenly, you're not just a parent, a leader, or a creative force, you are a patient.

This moment is called *identity rupture*, akin to an earthquake that splits you down the middle. It's one of the least-discussed consequences of a chronic diagnosis, yet it marks the exact point where your inner story fractures under the weight of a new reality.

As Viktor Frankl wrote from within the depths of suffering:

> *"Everything can be taken from a person but one thing: the last of the human freedoms, is to choose one's attitude in any given set of circumstances."*

In the face of uncertainty, the human spirit searches for continuity, looking for something to hold onto. But when your body fails you, and others begin relating to you differently, it's easy to internalize a new identity shaped by limitation.

This isn't a weakness. It's in the wiring. The mind naturally forms "I am" statements to make sense of the world:

> *"I am strong."* → *"I am sick."* → *"I am fading."*

This is where awareness becomes medicine. Recognizing that your identity is not fixed, but narrated and this decline in narration signfying the first step toward claiming your new identity.

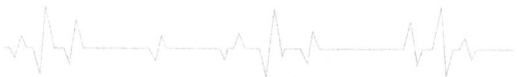

The Danger of the Label

Let's be honest: the label "patient" is seductive. It gives us structure. It explains why we're tired. It justifies the grief.

But it's also a trap.

This is where the Sapir-Whorf Hypothesis becomes relevant. In linguistics, it proposes that *the language we use not only describes reality, it limits how we perceive it.*

If you speak of yourself only as a patient, your world begins to shape around that role. Your power gets outsourced to doctors. Your identity becomes passive, reactive, even invisible.

You begin to shrink and retreat within your story.

What if, instead of saying "I am a patient," you said: *"I am a Titan."*?

Reclaiming the Narrative: Becoming a Titan

The word "Titan" might sound mythic, and to be honest, it's meant to.

In decoding philosophy, a Titan is not defined by the presence or absence of disease. A Titan is defined by the act of continuing to show up and grow despite a diagnosis.

> *A Titan is someone who rises from identity rupture and says: This is still my story to write.*

We do not deny the diagnosis. But we refuse to collapse into it.

To reclaim your narrative:

- Speak your identity aloud. "I am learning," "I am growing," "I am decoding."

- Journal from the I perspective. "I felt... I chose... I discovered..."

- Name your inner critic, as I did with "Charlie", to separate doubt from truth.

- Align with a symbol: a totem, a phrase, a memory of strength. Something that reminds you daily: I am more than what's been written about me.

This is the core of *The Knife Edge of Time:* rewriting the present, not repeating the past.

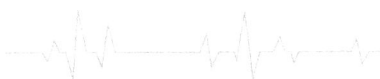

The Alignment of Identity

Just as illness touches Mind, Body, and Soul, so too does identity.

- **Mind Identity:** The thoughts and beliefs you hold about who you are.

- **Body Identity:** How you experience your form, its capacities, and limits.

- **Soul Identity:** The part of you that yearns for connection, meaning, and legacy.

Illness can distort any one of these, but healing requires bringing all three back into harmony. This is the beginning of dynamic identity realignment and it is foundational to your transformation.

Foreshadowing Reinvention

Healing is not about returning to who you were.

It's about *becoming* who you are meant to be.

This chapter is your first invitation to look beyond survival. To begin imagining reinvention. Here, now, on the *Knife Edge of Time*, you choose how to live, how to define, and how to become.

In the next chapter, we'll explore the structure beneath the philosophy of the Elements, Forces, and Harmony that shape your daily experience and help you begin building a more resilient, intentional future.

Key Insight

A chronic diagnosis can interrupt your story, but it doesn't get to end it. You do.

Practical Reflections

- Where have you unconsciously accepted an identity shaped by your diagnosis?

- What parts of your identity are most important to you and how can they guide your recovery?

- What does it mean for you to think, do, and act like a Titan today?

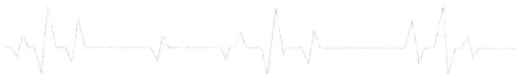

Fama's Sidebar

Rediscovering your identity through diagnosis might shift how others see you, but it doesn't have to change how you see yourself. You are still whole. Still you. Still capable of writing the next chapter. Even if today is a tough one, remind yourself: "I am more than this condition. I am choosing who I become.

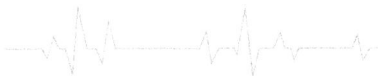

CHAPTER 5

Elements, Forces & Dynamic Harmony

At the outset of my heart disease diagnosis, I was in a denial daze.

Outwardly, I maintained a "business as usual" front, but inside, I was teetering on the edge of despair. My prognosis was severe, and every indicator suggested further decline. However, I knew from my prostate disease journey that waiting for things to get worse wasn't an option.

Thankfully I had my *Foundation Stone* to call upon as a structured record of my chronic past, containing everything I had learned about my health history. From that foundation I surmised future success meant stabilizing my heart health through nutrition, structured movement, and stress reduction techniques, all while closely monitoring my physical and emotional state.

For a while, it worked. The condition remained steady. But months later, my heart crash changed everything. My health plummeted from stability to catastrophic decline in weeks. If I didn't act fast, I wasn't going to make it.

With all that hindsight, I was still missing something.

My wife recognized what I couldn't: I was spiraling into depression. At her urging, I sought mental health therapy, which led me to revisit my old recovery notes from prostate cancer. Those notes became the foundation for something bigger, a complete approach that would later form *Decode Your Diagnosis*.

I realized that tackling the condition required more than just physical adjustments, I needed to take control of my entire existence. That meant:

- Understanding my commitments and stressors.

- Rethinking my nutrition and exercise from the ground up.

- Adding mental and emotional resilience strategies, including journaling and guided reflection.

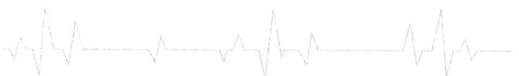

This holistic approach wasn't just about survival; it was about reclaiming my future. And it started with a single decision; to fight back.

Within weeks, my heart health stabilized, and in just a few months, I saw an incredible recovery from the lowest heart health of 42% to the highest result since the original diagnosis of 83%, all in under three months.

Decoding your diagnosis begins with a simple but profound truth. Your life is not defined by a single diagnosis, a single treatment, or even a single part of you. It is shaped by the dynamic interplay of three essential facets. *The elements* that make you, *the forces* you encounter both within and around you and the constant balance of flux these facets seek as dynamic harmony.

It is here, in the dance between Elements, Forces and the pursuit of Dynamic Harmony, that the true journey of decoding your diagnosis begins.

The Decoding Facets: Elements, Forces, and Dynamic Harmony

Let's explore some foundational concepts of the Framework and how they can apply to you.

Your life is shaped by three interrelated facets: Elements, Forces, and Harmony. Together, they provide a lens for understanding where you are and what steps you can take to move toward *Functional Integrity*.

- **Elements:** The internal foundation of who you are is your Mind, Body, and Soul. These are the personal dimensions of your being, interconnected and dynamic.

- **Forces:** The external influences that act upon your Elements. Environment, lifestyle, stress, and time are all examples of Forces that shape your health and well-being.

- **Dynamic Harmony:** The balance you strive to achieve between internal Elements and external Forces. Dynamic Harmony is not static; it's an ongoing dance, adapting to life's constant changes.

Understanding these facets offers a roadmap for navigating your diagnosis. It helps you see how internal and external factors have brought you to this point and how realignment is possible.

I first understood the true power of decoding when I began working with my mental health professional in the early months of my heart disease diagnosis.

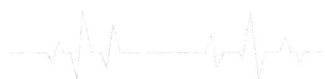

Around the same time, I read *Solve for Happy* by Mo Gawdat, which introduced me to the idea of naming my inner critic. Following his lead, I gave mine a name, Charlie. I thought I could fix my body while ignoring the emotional and spiritual toll the condition was taking. I was wrong.

My clinician helped me see that my mind and soul were just as critical to recovery as my body. Together, we worked on my elements:

1. **Mind:** Learning to challenge the force of my inner critic (Charlie) and replace self-doubt with constructive reflection.

2. **Body:** Implementing structured, sustainable exercise and nutrition habits that supported my heart health rather than impact it.

3. **Soul:** Rediscovering passion through writing, meditation, and reframing setbacks as opportunities.

Elements

Let's explore the facets of decoding your diagnosis individually so you can apply them to your own situation starting with the Elements.

The Elements are the essence of your being. They represent your Mind, your Body, and your Soul, collectively they become the interconnected parts that define you as a whole.

Each Element influences the others, creating a dynamic interplay that reflects your overall well-being and while you could fill a library with the books written about each of these topics, here's a short summary of the key characteristics of the three elements.

- **Mind**
  Your mental state is the control center for your actions and decisions. Chronic stress, for example, can create a mental loop of fear and worry, preventing you from seeing solutions. Conversely, a growth-focused mindset can open doors to positive change.

- **Body**
  Your physical state is a mirror of your habits, environment, and lifestyle. Pain, fatigue, or illness are not signs of failure; they are messages urging you to pay attention and realign. Your Body is your most tangible Element, yet it is deeply interconnected with your Mind and Soul.

- **Soul**
  Your Soul is about connection and meaning. It encompasses the things that give your life purpose such as relationships, creativity, community, or the quiet joy of presence. A nurtured Soul fuels resilience and fulfillment, while a neglected Soul can lead to emptiness.

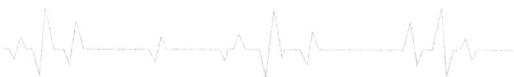

Forces

While the Elements are internal, Forces represent the external influences that shape your life. These Forces act on your Mind, Body, and Soul, sometimes pushing them into alignment, other times pulling them out of balance.

- **Environment**
  Your surroundings have a profound impact on your well-being. A supportive environment can buffer stress, while a toxic one can exacerbate strain.

- **Lifestyle**
  Choices in nutrition, exercise, and sleep either support or challenge your health. Small, consistent changes in lifestyle habits can create significant shifts.

- **Stress and Time**
  Chronic stress drains your resources, while poor time management traps you in unsustainable patterns.

Dynamic Harmony

Dynamic Harmony is the equilibrium you strive for when your internal Elements align with external Forces. It's not about achieving perfection; it's about creating a flow that adapts to life's demands while maintaining your center.

- **Dynamic Equilibrium:** Harmony isn't about eliminating stress but about learning to flow with it, like grass bending in the wind.

- **The Fallacy of Balance:** True Harmony acknowledges life's motion. The key is to remain flexible and intentional, adjusting to support your alignment.

Life as an Interconnected Web

Let's reflect on how the core facets of decoding your diagnosis come into play.

Life isn't a sequence of isolated events or unrelated pieces. It's a dynamic, interconnected web where every decision, action, and experience shapes the whole. This perspective lies at the heart of decoding your diagnosis, representing a model for resilience and growth that integrates your Mind, Body, and Soul.

By viewing yourself as a unified system rather than a collection of parts, you can align these *elements*, adapt to external forces, and create *dynamic harmony* amidst life's challenges. This process is not about perfection but about cultivating resilience, adaptability, and balance.

Decode Your Diagnosis draws from two profound sources:

- **Modern Science's Systems View of Life:** Thinkers like Fritjof Capra emphasize that life thrives on relationships and feedback loops. Every system, whether an ecosystem, a family, or a person, is shaped by constant interactions.

- **Ancient Philosophy of Harmony:** The Taoist concept of Yin and Yang sees life as a balance of dynamic forces, where health arises from adapting to and balancing these influences.

By combining these perspectives, Decode Your Diagnosis offers a practical framework for understanding yourself as a whole, dynamic being. It provides a pathway for navigating life's complexities while cultivating *Functional Integrity*, where all parts of your being, and the interventions you employ, work together in harmony.

Decoding isn't a checklist, it isn't a one-time exercise. It's a constant recalibration, a life long practice of awareness, adjustment and action.

As we explore the Mind, Body, and Soul, think of each Element as a pillar supporting your foundation. When one pillar falters, the others must adapt to maintain stability. Your goal is not perfection but *Dynamic Harmony*; an ongoing balance that allows your Alignment to thrive amidst life's changes.

Key Insight

Your health is shaped by more than one system or symptom because it's the relationship between your elements, impacting your Mind, Body, and Soul, and how you respond to the Forces around you that creates true healing.

Practical Reflections

The Alignment Workbook
It's never too late to download the *Alignment Workbook* from our website if you haven't already, I suggest you do it from the following link:

decodeyourdiagnosis.com

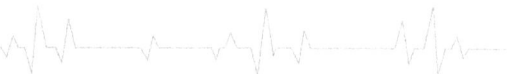

Elements

What's one area of your Mind, Body, or Soul that you've neglected recently and how could you begin to nurture it?

Forces

Which external Force has had the greatest impact on your health lately and what would it look like to reduce its pressure?

Dynamic Harmony

Think of a moment when you felt grounded and aligned. What helped you get there, and what could help you return?

Fama Sidebar: The Navigator's Insight

Reflection of what's impacting you is your first tool. By exploring your Elements, Forces, and Harmony, you're learning the map of your journey.

CHAPTER 6

Exploring Your Elements

I was walking through Suva city in Fiji, days after the heart disease diagnosis. My fitness level at the time was relatively high and walking was something I did quite a lot when visiting international cities to keep my physical health in peak shape for the rigours of international business. I remember the day quite clearly. I was walking between a meeting with the Minister for Infrastructure and my next one with the Fijian Chamber of Commerce and Industry.

To fill time I rang the Chair of the corporation I worked for back in Australia to advise him of my fresh diagnosis with CAD and CSVD. The call itself was rather matter of fact, even procedural to be honest, but the moment after I hung up I needed to stop and sit under a Betel Nut tree to gather my composure. When I say 'gather my composure', I'm talking all out emotional upheaval culminating it terse words being shouted at the defenceless tree and a healthy dose of crying, not in pity of my diagnosis, but in drawing a line in the sand of my life long career.

I was fractured. My body felt quite fine, I was fit, I ate healthily, yet my mind and soul were smashed. This wasn't my first rodeo with a chronic condition but it was the first one to impact my career. That feeling of my career disappearing under my feet was as real as standing under a shower. Work life, as I came to enjoy it, would be over. In addition, part of my recommendation was to reduce travel and refrain from dangerous environments like my sojourns to Papua New Guinea. Danger was what I did for a living and I cherished the opportunities of doing business on the frontier of humanity.

But, in that short phone call I had personally called a halt to that life, I knew at that moment, that I had voluntarily kickstarted the demise of my professional career and I was shattered. That moment under the Betel Nut tree was the starting gate of internal struggle between my three elements. What started as a subtle moment became all out brutal competition for my limited personal resources.

My mind was having a field day, with Charlie running wild, playing with my emotions and encouraging thoughts of the apocalypse. As far as Charlie was concerned, I was doomed.

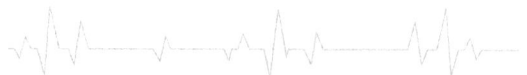

My body refused to give up its dominance as the stoic survivor. Fitness had to be maintained, or the wheels of civilisation would definitely fall off. So I did more laps in whatever pool I could find, and I walked extra kilometers every day, with my watch dutifully coaching me toward continuous improvement.

Again, if I'm brutally honest I had no idea my Soul even existed at this stage. As far as my capitalist self knew. The Soul was some wu wu approach to religion so my spirituality just got left behind entirely.

The breaking point of my internal struggle with the diagnosis happened when I was back home in Australia. I was a few months into the CAD/ CSVD diagnosis and I began to get aggravated easily and that's when my wife gently stepped in suggesting I needed to talk to someone about my mental health. I talk about this in more detail elsewhere, but my point is, the moment felt like a strategic failure indicating that the focus on my physical health without addressing my mental health was patently floored and the single-element approach collapsed when I called a psychologist and we explored the root cause of my dilemma.

The physical fitness had to continue to facilitate mental and spiritual rehabilitation but it was clear a functionally integrated approach was necessary to uplift all my elements.

As the subject of my own survival, I had to acknowledge each element had it's own truth and somehow I had to give all three of them an equal voice if I was to have an empowered diagnosis.

For mental health, I became a student, working with my psychologist, doing my homework and constantly keeping Charlie in check. As time and my mental skill set improved, I even became the subject of my own personal experiment exploring split personality traits. For my body I became the PT coach actively championing the efforts of my training and researching a life plan focused on coronary conditions. As much as I tried in those first twelve months I still couldn't identify what it meant to let my Soul express itself. I took my psychologist's advice and started immersing myself in creativity writing this book, and that felt really good, but I still didn't have a sense of self, an identity for the future, so rather than beating myself up I decided to let it ride for a while knowing I would give it due focus when the more pressing concerns with my mental health had been resolved.

When it came to matters of the Soul I really had to nurture it as you would a neglected personal relationship because, it had to take a back seat while I focused on the more pressing issues of Mental Health.

Healing the Soul meant starting with the basics and taking a keen interest in spirituality from as many cultural traditions as I could find. Everything from the Abrahamic religions we all know, to more specialised teachings such as Heartfulness Yoga and Daoist philosophy.

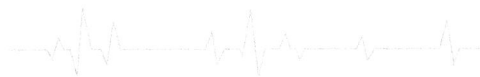

Taking it even further, my wife and I became dual Pilgrims together, hiking the Unesco listed path of the Kumano Kodo in Japan. While on this journey of enlightenment, we experienced the tranquility and spirituality of the Three Grand Shinto Shrines of Kumano trekking through mountainous landscapes, lush forests and experiencing traditional village hospitality. This spiritual immersion peaked when we participated in the buddhist Jukai ceremony while sleeping amongst the temples of Koyasan, the origin of Japanese Buddhism.

While I am constantly seeking alignment across the Elements, it's not often you feel true harmony with all three, but I had experienced it after my return from our Heartfulness retreat in India. Sure, you might say it was a flow on effect from two weeks of deep immersion in Yogic philosophy and meditation, but it was real and was like pure harmony. My body was tracking consistently well, my mind was clear, even Charlie was silent and for the first time since diagnosis, I knew where I was heading spiritually for my future self. I knew the future me I wanted to become. In that moment I could see exactly who my future self was.

I suppose the best way to explain the feeling was like creating a strategic team plan that you present to your group and the weeks afterward it all falls into place and you experience the rare moment when everyone is in alignment.

This was the first taste of what was possible in my future and with that I now know what to practice on and where alignment can be found. In a way, it's about honouring my decoding not just as individual elements but as a collective whole that when aligned take you to a level free of diagnosis, free of unnecessary fear and hurt.

Honouring yourself is an interesting concept and one that often gets confused with self-aggrandizement, so no, honour is not about standing on a pedestal it's about staying as humble as a warrior monk and treating yourself as a complex living system not something to splash on socials with a selfie.

Am I always humble, of course not but I am always aiming to honour the three elements of my personal Trinity.

A diagnosis doesn't just affect your body. It reverberates through your entire being, your thoughts, your emotions, and your sense of self. In Decode Your Diagnosis, we call these interconnected aspects your Elements: Mind, Body, and Soul. They are not isolated systems; they are dynamically linked. When one is impacted, all respond. Healing and resilience arise from understanding and aligning these Elements as a lived experience, not just a philosophical concept.

Let's now explore each one with practical insight, not as abstract categories, but as active parts of your daily life.

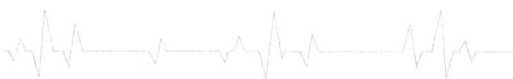

Mind: The Architect of Thought

The mind isn't just where thought happens, it's where stories are formed, identities are shaped, and decisions are made. After a diagnosis, the mind can become a battleground of what-ifs, fears, and self-doubt. But it can also be your greatest ally in the journey toward resilience.

You don't need to silence negative thoughts to reclaim mental alignment, you need to reframe them. The goal is not to eliminate fear but to face it with clarity. When you practice gratitude, mindful breathing, or journaling from the "I" perspective, you create space between reaction and intention. This is how you train the mind to support your healing rather than hinder it.

Body: The Foundation of Experience

Your body is your frontline in the journey with chronic illness. It sends signals, pain, fatigue, inflammation, to alert you when something is off. The body doesn't just carry your condition; it reflects how you live.

Learning to listen to your body without judgment is one of the most powerful practices you can adopt. Hydration, movement, sleep, nutrition, these aren't checklists. They're daily conversations. When you learn what energizes you, what drains you, and how your body responds to change, you gain insight into your own operating manual. Alignment here means tuning into those signals and adjusting accordingly.

Soul: The Compass of Meaning

The soul is often overlooked in conventional medicine, but it is essential to Functional Integrity. It's the part of you that asks, "Why does this matter?" It seeks connection, meaning, and legacy. Chronic illness can cause you to feel disconnected from who you were, but your soul reminds you who you are becoming.

Cultivating the soul doesn't require a religious practice, but it does demand reflection. Rhetorically, What brings you joy? What relationships nourish you? What stories do you want to tell? Whether it's through creativity, nature, service, or stillness, tending to the soul adds depth and direction to your healing journey.

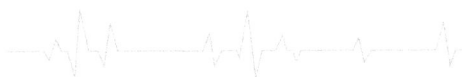

The Interplay of the Three

These elements don't exist in isolation. They inform and influence each other constantly. Mental stress affects sleep and digestion. Poor nutrition dulls clarity. Lack of purpose deflates energy. But the reverse is also true:

- A calm mind supports better physical outcomes.

- A nourished body fosters emotional steadiness.

- A purposeful soul strengthens your will to act.

To explore your Elements is to map your terrain. The more familiar you become with their signals, the more equipped you are to navigate change with confidence.

Key Insight

Mind, Body, and Soul are not abstract categories. They are active, lived elements of your daily experience. When aligned, they form the foundation of your resilience.

Practical Reflections

- When have you noticed your mind, body, and soul falling out of sync?

- What was the result?

- What daily practices help each of your Elements feel acknowledged and supported?

- Which of the three Elements feels most neglected right now?
  a.   What is one step you can take to re-engage with it?

Fama's Sidebar

Listen for the signals your Elements are always speaking. The tension in your shoulders, the spark of joy, the restless thoughts at 3am, these are messages. Don't ignore them. Learn to listen. That's where real alignment begins.

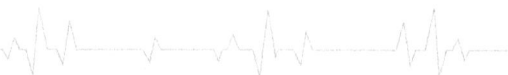

CHAPTER 7

The Forces At Play

For me, the early stages of heart disease and cancer, post-diagnosis were somewhat of a false start. Life went on, because the first stage of grief is denial, so I continued on from that first outpouring under the Betel Nut tree. Maintaining my stoic composure, like executives should, it was business as usual.

Silently however, my mind and body had a difference of opinion and it took a good two to three months for cracks to appear because during that time I still had a corporate role to up keep, it was christmas time with family and work stresses like quarterly board reports still had to be done and then there were rounds of medical analysis to undergo.

As the true extent of my condition began to be clear, the cracks began to appear.

The cracks first surfaced in my temperament and then migrated out into my personality and that's when my wife politely guided me towards mental health therapy. All of a sudden I went from being an extrovert to being insular, defensive and introverted.

I just wasn't my normal self and it began to show in my personal relationships with my family, at work and a general level of pessimism crept in. One thing I remember internally grappling with was the suggestion I had three to five years life expectancy. When I told people the extent of my condition they nearly always gasped.

I thought if I increased my exercise I could reduce stress. My wife and I hadn't drunk alcohol for over five years, our diet was quite healthy but we turned that up a notch as well switching to primarily pescatarian with the occasional lean meat.

No matter how much I worked on my body, things just didn't seem to improve, my personality continued to decline.

The 'aha' moment came during the first therapy session with my psychologist. The realisation I was going through grief and although I didn't understand the depth of depression I was in, the layers of the onion we needed to work on became evidently clear.

And look, he was a great clinician so he didn't load me up but I could see from the nature of the discussion that we needed quite a bit of work if I was to have any chance of decoding my diagnosis.

The thing I didn't understand so well was the level of impact stress had on me as a force both mentally and physically. I mean, if you want someone to manage a serious crisis like a multimillion dollar project being destroyed by a cyclone, I'm your man, and yes I was leading an organisation when that actually happened. In fact Cyclone Yasi's attack on our business was actually the third worst thing that happened to our organisation that disaster season, but the company, my family and I came through it.

What I am only now coming to understand is that the ability to weather 'stress storms' impacts me heavily internally, both mentally and physically.

When I think back to the years of external forces I've shouldered during prostate disease and heart disease, by 'managing stress well', I wonder how I'm even still alive.

The real shift or realignment began roughly six months after the first mental therapy intervention. I reflect on that year as having two functional halves of personal growth. The first part working through the grief of diagnosis and the second half in realigning myself toward life as a Titan decoding their diagnosis.

I tell you, that second half was quite a relief, not just for me but also those around me.

How can I describe it... Ok, try holding a really deep breath until you start gagging for oxygen and then release it and think how you feel directly after you've taken your next breath. Go on, try it now and see how you feel. Feel that immense relief.

Got it, great, now picture yourself as I was in the early stages of our marriage when my wife and I were out on a diving voyage and I snorkelled down 25 meters (75 feet) to retrieve the skippers favourite filleting knife I had accidently dropped over the side. I was a diving instructor at the time, so I could hold my breath pretty well and the visibility was crystal clear, so I could see the shimmer of the knife from the surface. Not one to shy away from a challenge, off I went over the side without telling anyone I was gone, down, down, down and... got ya. The knife and I slowly returned to the surface and in those last few meters before reaching the surface I started blacking out due to hypoxia. If you think the relief you felt when you took that breath was lovely, imagine the desperate exhilaration I felt upon taking my first breath when I smashed through the surface on that free dive.

That level of desperate exhilaration is how I felt midway through the second half of the diagnosis year, when I began offloading non essential stress. The biggest single act or event was the day I stood down from my executive roles. The levity this act produced to my overall condition was incredible. I suddenly felt I had a future.

Now, eight months further on and I'm a renewed, revitalised me. I won't say I'm a different person because we are who we are because of all we have experienced, not a new someone because of it.

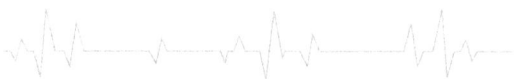

The biggest change to who I am is how I manage everything in life, from stress to enjoying the knife edge of time. It's like I'm surfing waves. The thing about surfing is it's ability to hold you in the moment. There is nothing else, once you catch that wave, every part of your being is focused on riding that wave, there is no other way to stay on your board than engulf yourself in the moment. Life is like that for me now. At the moment I am passionately engrossed in writing this story and enjoying the sculpting of every word and shortly, I'll be walking away from the keyboard and turning to riding by bicycle into town. Whether it's washing dishes, doing exercises or practicing meditation. If I'm doing something, I'm riding that wave 100%.

One thing I have come to understand is how to reduce stress by recognising a force and letting it pass like water off a duck's back. Where once I would try to counter a force, now I flow with it and the outcome is vastly different and I feel so much better for it as well.

Now I'm living the life of a Titan.

A diagnosis doesn't arrive in a vacuum. It arrives in a context shaped by your history, your habits, your surroundings, and your stress levels. These shaping influences, both subtle and strong, are what we refer to in Decode Your Diagnosis as *Forces*.

If the Elements (Mind, Body, and Soul) are the internal landscape of your being, then the Forces are the winds, waves, and weather that act upon that landscape. Understanding these Forces, and learning how to navigate them, is the key to building Dynamic Harmony.

The Two Categories of Force

Forces can be divided into two primary types:

1. **External Forces** — These are the environmental, social, and situational pressures that influence your Elements. They include:
   • Physical environment (pollution, housing, noise, nature access)
   • Social influences (relationships, support networks, media exposure)
   • Professional or economic pressure (job demands, financial strain)
   • Life events (grief, trauma, celebration, caregiving roles)

2. **Internal Forces** — These arise from within and directly impact how you interpret and respond to the world. They include:
   • Beliefs and mindset
   • Emotional regulation
   • Habits and routines
   • Your inner critic or personal narrative

External Forces often trigger Internal Forces. For example, the stress of a demanding job (external) may activate self-doubt or perfectionism (internal). That's why awareness matters because not all Forces are visible.

How Forces Shape The Decoding Process

Each Force has a directional impact. It can:

- Align your Elements
  (e.g., time in nature improves both mood and immune function).
- Disrupt your Elements
  (e.g., social conflict drains mental energy and creates physical tension).
- Mask disharmony
  (e.g., numbing with alcohol or overworking to avoid discomfort).

The goal isn't to eliminate Forces, that's impossible. Instead, we learn to:

- Observe them.
- Understand their source.
- Choose how to respond.

The Role of Time and Stress

Two Forces deserve special attention:

- **Time** is a neutral Force that becomes either supportive or destructive depending on how it's used.
  - Poor time management increases stress and reduces space for rest and recovery.
  - Good time management reduces stress and offers space for life to flow in it's natural rhythm.
- **Stress** is a compound Force that amplifies others. Chronic stress affects the nervous system, immune response, cognition, and emotional balance. It's not the presence of stress that harms us, it's the lack of recalibration.

That's where Dynamic Harmony becomes your tool of transformation.

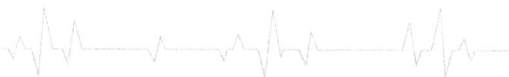

Introducing Force Mapping

Force Mapping is a reflective tool. It's a method of identifying and evaluating the key Forces acting on your Elements.

Ask yourself:

- What's pressing in on me lately?
- What supports me right now?
- Are there recurring patterns or triggers?
- Which Forces are within my influence to shift?

Mapping these Forces helps create clarity. Clarity leads to action.

Force Interplay in Daily Life

Here's how Forces commonly interact with the Elements:

- A **toxic work environment** (external) may lead to anxiety (Mind), tension (Body), and loss of purpose (Soul).
- **Unprocessed grief** (internal) may lead to isolation (Soul), insomnia (Body), and negative self-talk (Mind).
- **Supportive relationships** can buffer difficult experiences, helping to maintain equilibrium across all three Elements.

This is why addressing only one Element rarely works. Forces don't respect boundaries. They cascade.

Empowerment Through Awareness

Recognizing the Forces at play is the beginning of choice. You may not control the weather, but you can choose what to wear, when to rest, and how to build shelter.

The same goes for your journey. With awareness comes adaptability. With adaptability comes resilience. And with resilience comes the ability to decode your diagnosis, not through perfection, but through intentional alignment.

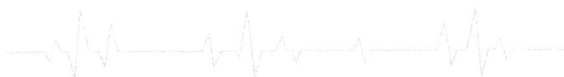

Key Insight

Forces are ever-present, but they don't have to dictate your direction. Awareness gives you power. Response gives you freedom.

Practical Reflections

• What's one Force, either internal or external, that has impacted your health journey recently?

• How has it influenced your Mind, Body, and Soul?

• What's one shift (however small) you can make to respond with intention?

Fama's Sidebar

Be the Observer. Not every storm needs to be fought. Some need to be watched, understood, and navigated around. Let awareness be your compass. Before you react, pause and notice the Force. Then choose your next step with clarity.

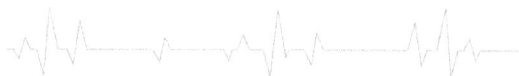

CHAPTER 8

Practicing Dynamic Harmony

Dynamic Harmony plays a vital role in reducing stress and supporting long-term health within Decode Your Diagnosis. Because of its wide-reaching impact, it deserves a chapter dedicated entirely to its exploration.

What Is Dynamic Harmony?

Before we go any further let's reflect on its definition. Dynamic Harmony is the interplay between your internal Elements (Mind, Body, Soul) and external Forces. It's the ongoing process of recognizing shifts in your environment, and within yourself, and responding with intention to maintain alignment.

At its core, Dynamic Harmony is about awareness and action. Awareness helps you identify when one Element is out of sync, and action gives you the power to realign. This practice acknowledges that life is fluid, and true resilience lies in the ability to adapt gracefully to changes, setbacks, and growth opportunities.

For example, imagine you are managing chronic fatigue (Body) while also feeling emotionally disconnected from loved ones (Soul). Dynamic Harmony would prompt you to observe these signals, explore their causes, and take intentional steps such as adjusting your physical activities and prioritizing quality time with supportive relationships to restore some resemblance of balance.

Let me clarify that we're not striving for balance in the traditional sense. Dynamic Harmony is not 'balance' because balance is a momentary concept that is not sustainable. Think back to your childhood and how hard it was to get that sea-saw to stop in the middle with both sides level, and when it finally did, the slightest movement saw it quickly fall to one side or the other. Come forward into adulthood and the classic example most of us have considered at some time in our lives, work-life balance. If you found that then you are an amazing unicorn.

For these very reasons, while travelling your *Alignment Pathway* always aim for dynamic harmony, not balance.

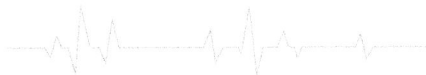

Practical Steps to Cultivate Dynamic Harmony

Recognizing the Signals

Dynamic Harmony begins with awareness by paying attention to the cues your Mind, Body, and Soul are sending. These might include:

- **Emotional Signals:** Stress, irritability, or lack of motivation.

- **Physical Signals:** Fatigue, tension, or disrupted sleep.

- **Spiritual Signals:** Feeling disconnected from purpose or joy.

By learning to identify these signals early during the prostate disease diagnosis, I was able to take proactive steps to address them. After repeatedly pushing myself to try and engage my previous identity, prior to the cancer, I realised it would be impossible, that I was being too hard on myself and suffering the consequences. Once I acknowledged the fact that I couldn't turn back, and accepted I would wear incontinence pads and be impotent, I started to set the main concerns aside and identify subtle signs before they escalated:

- **Mental strain:** When I felt "uptight" before full-blown stress, I knew it was time to increase meditation (yes, meditation not medication, hehehe).

- **Physical fatigue:** The first twinges of exhaustion meant I had to cap my daily physical exertion at two hours.

- **Spiritual unrest:** If I felt disconnected, I'd dedicate extra reflection time to recalibrating my sense of purpose.

These small adjustments prevented me from hitting major crashes and allowed me to sustain long-term progress.

Recalibrating Through Action

Once I'd recognized misalignment, the next step was taking intentional action to restore balance. It's important to start small and focus on one Element at a time.

- **Mind:** Practice mindfulness exercises, like deep breathing or gratitude journaling.

- **Body:** Prioritize hydration, balanced meals, or gentle movement.

- **Soul:** Engage in activities that bring joy or connect you to your values, such as art, nature, or meaningful conversations.

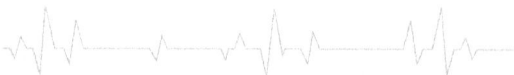

Recalibrating isn't about overhauling everything at once, it's about making strategic, small adjustments to regain stability.

For example, there was a time during the early stages of my heart disease diagnosis when I noticed my deep sleep quality declining and research into deep sleep suggests this is the time when the body repairs. I definitely needed to allow my body to repair so it was then I decided it was time to seriously recalibrate my lifestyle to improve sleep by:

- **Adjusting bedtime:** By returning to a sleep schedule that focused on natural biorhythms for deep sleep, by moving forward lights-out to 9:00PM – 9:30 PM and wearing eye masks and meditating before sleep to flush the mind.

- **Shifting meal timing:** Following the "eat breakfast like a king, lunch like a prince, dinner like a pauper" principle reduced digestion interference.

- **Eliminating caffeine and sugar after 3 PM:** This small change dramatically improved sleep depth.

By making these targeted adjustments, I was able to restore my sleep quality to over 90%, ensuring my body could properly repair and recover.

Building a Supportive Environment

It requires surrounding yourself with people, tools, and practices that reinforce your wellbeing. While future chapters will explore some of these resources in detail, what's essential right now is recognizing the value of support and beginning to shape an environment that sustains your growth.

Sustaining Dynamic Harmony isn't just about personal habits. It's about aligning your surroundings and relationships with your goals so that your progress is supported, not sabotaged.

A classic example of the power of your support network came in my first year with CAD, I struggled to balance career ambitions with health needs. I was still trying to prove I could do it all, even though stress was actively working against my recovery.

The turning point? Unwavering support from my wife.

She was there when I had to make the hard decisions, like stepping down from my CEO role and rethinking long-term professional commitments. Her steady presence helped me navigate one of the most difficult transitions of my life.

A strong support network is invaluable. Having at least one person who understands your goals and holds you accountable can make all the difference.

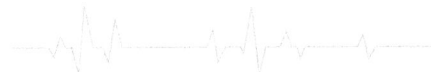

Creating a Daily Realignment Routine

Incorporate small daily rituals to maintain alignment. For example:

- Morning check-ins: Spend 5 minutes reflecting on what your decoding needs today.

- Evening gratitude: Note one way you practiced Dynamic Harmony during the day.

- Before bed: offload your thoughts into your journal for future reference.

The Role of Joy in Dynamic Harmony

One of the most overlooked aspects of maintaining Dynamic Harmony is the role of joy. For years, I believed that my health journey was about discipline, structure, and sacrifice. What I failed to recognize was that without joy, sustainability is impossible.

I realized this when I noticed how much energy I had after engaging in activities that genuinely brought me happiness like listening to music, writing, and even rewatching classic films from my youth. These weren't just hobbies; they were key contributors to my well-being.

I started applying this principle in practical ways:

- Instead of rigidly sticking to a set fitness routine, I introduced long walks in the bush that felt natural and restorative.

- Rather than just focusing on nutrition from a health perspective, I began cooking meals that brought me comfort as well.

- I allowed myself to laugh more, engage socially, and prioritize joy as a fundamental part of my daily routine.

What I discovered was profound: joy is regenerative. It acts as a natural counterbalance to stress, helping to restore the energy we expend managing our health. Without it, burnout is inevitable.

True Dynamic Harmony isn't about perfection, it's about ensuring that Mind, Body, and Soul are all nourished, including through joy. Recognizing the importance of happiness in my health journey transformed not just my outlook but my ability to sustain long-term well-being.

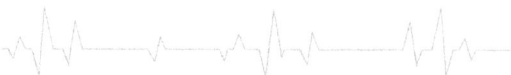

The Art of Balance

Dynamic Harmony isn't about achieving a perfect balance, it's about developing the flexibility to realign when life pulls you in different directions. For Titans navigating a diagnosis, this concept is especially critical. Life will throw unexpected Forces at you, and Dynamic Harmony helps you adapt, pivot, and thrive amidst the chaos.

By integrating your Mind, Body, and Soul with the Forces of life, you can cultivate resilience and growth, even in the face of adversity. Unlike rigid perfectionism, Dynamic Harmony embraces the unpredictability of life, offering a framework for continuous recalibration.

Exploring Dynamic Harmony

The Role of Reflection

Dynamic Harmony operates through regular self reflection. These reflections after we experience changes resulting from feedback loops when one Element compensates for another, creating signals that something needs attention. For example:

- **Emotional Signals:** Feelings of overwhelm or irritability might suggest your Mind is overloaded and could benefit from mindfulness practices or breaks.

- **Physical Signals:** Persistent fatigue or muscle tension may indicate a need to reassess your Body's needs, such as sleep or nutrition.

- **Spiritual Signals:** A sense of emptiness or lack of direction may highlight the need to reconnect with your Soul's purpose.

Feedback loops serve as reminders to pause, reflect, and adjust. The sooner you recognize these signals, the easier it becomes to make small, meaningful changes before imbalance escalates.

Dynamic Harmony vs. Perfectionism

One common misconception is that achieving harmony means maintaining a perfect balance at all times. In reality, Dynamic Harmony is the opposite of perfectionism. It's about flexibility, not rigidity; growth, not stagnation.

Consider a tightrope walker: their goal isn't to stand still but to keep moving forward while making constant micro-adjustments. In the same way, Dynamic Harmony teaches you to embrace imperfection and focus on progress rather than unrealistic ideals.

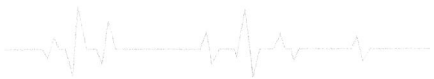

The Role of Flexibility

Dynamic Harmony is supported through maintaining flexibility and encouraging adaptability, intention, and self-reflection.

Adaptability
Adaptability is the ability to adjust your actions, expectations, and mindset in response to changing circumstances. It's what allows you to pivot when life doesn't go as planned.
 • Example: If your usual fitness routine becomes unsustainable due to a flare-up, adaptability might mean finding gentler activities like yoga or stretching to stay active without overexertion.

Intention
Intention is about acting with purpose, even when life feels chaotic. It's the anchor that keeps your adjustments aligned with your values and goals.
 • Example: When work demands increase, intention helps you prioritize family dinners or self-care rituals to maintain connection and resilience.

Self-Reflection
Self-reflection is the practice of regularly checking in with the process of decoding Mind, Body & Soul to identify what needs attention and how to recalibrate. It allows you to track patterns, recognize misalignment, and celebrate progress.
 • Example: Journaling about your energy levels or emotions can reveal trends that help you make informed adjustments to your routine.

Embracing the Flow

Dynamic Harmony is the art of living in alignment with your decoding amidst the ebb and flow of life. It's not about striving for a perfect balance but about cultivating the awareness, flexibility, and intention to adapt as needed.

By integrating the principles of Dynamic Harmony into your daily life, you can build resilience, foster growth, and navigate your Pathway with confidence and grace. Remember, the goal isn't to stop life's waves but to learn how to ride them with purpose and poise.

Now that you've learned how to listen to your inner compass and shift with life's tides, it's time to explore the deeper rhythm that governs your journey: time. In the next chapter, we'll introduce you to the Knife Edge Of Time as a way of living intentionally on the Knife Edge of Time, where your past informs your growth, your present anchors your actions, and your future draws you forward with purpose.

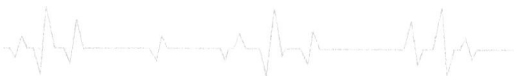

Key Insight

Dynamic Harmony is not about achieving balance, it's about adapting with awareness and intention when life shifts. Progress is the goal, not perfection.

Practical Reflections

Signals
- What recent emotional, physical, or spiritual signal has stood out to you?

Recalibration
- What is one small change you could make today to realign your energy across Mind, Body, or Soul?

Joy
- When was the last time you felt joy and with that in mind, what activity could you introduce or reintroduce into your life that feels deeply nourishing?

Fama's Sidebar: Embracing the Flow

Dynamic Harmony isn't about getting everything perfect, it's about learning to adjust when life shifts unexpectedly. Think of it like sailing a boat: you can't control the wind, but you can adjust your sails. The signals your Mind, Body, and Soul send to you are like a compass, guiding you to recalibrate when needed.

CHAPTER 9

Embracing The Knife Edge Of Time

When my heart crash occurred, it would have been easy to fall into despair. But I drew strength from a fundamental truth: I *had faced adversity before and came out stronger.*

Reflecting on my prostate disease and cancer journey, I saw how resilience was built through incremental progress. I didn't just wake up one day stronger, I fought for it. The same principle applied to my heart disease recovery. I journaled past successes, noting what had worked, what hadn't, and where my mindset needed to shift.

By acknowledging my past resilience, I reaffirmed my ability to navigate the present with confidence.

During my heart crash recovery, I realized that the present moment is where real change happens. I could plan for the future and reflect on the past, but action had to be taken now.

I implemented the following techniques to anchor myself in the present:

- **Daily Reflection:** I asked myself, *What is one thing I can do today that my future self will thank me for?*

- **Micro-Wins:** Instead of waiting for big achievements, I celebrated small victories like being able to walk an extra kilometer, embracing a moment of peace during meditation, or becoming engrossed in a good conversation.

- **Breath Awareness:** I practiced deep breathing techniques to re-center whenever I felt overwhelmed by taking three deep breaths. A simple but powerful tool to pause time and reconnect with the moment.

The more I focused on the present as a place of power, the more I saw progress unfold naturally.

If the past is a library, the future is a blank canvas, a space where dreams, aspirations, and possibilities reside. The future inspires, but it can also overwhelm. How do I plan a life around a diagnosis? How do I set goals when uncertainty looms?

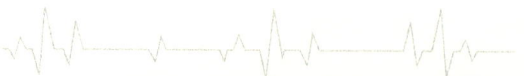

The Knife Edge Of Time encouraged me to approach the future with hope and intentionality. The key was found in setting goals that provided direction while remaining adaptable to the unexpected. Rather than fearing what lay ahead, I utilised the possibilities of the future as motivation to take deliberate and meaningful steps in the present.

The future is an incredible place to focus, but it can also be overwhelming. Early in my diagnosis, I struggled with thoughts of limitation like what if I never regained my health? What if my prognosis didn't improve?

Instead of dwelling on uncertainty, I set clear milestones, landing on achievable markers to guide my journey forward:

- Improve my heart health by 10% in six months.
- Walk 10,000 steps a day for at least four days per week.
- Strengthen my mental resilience through daily meditation.

Each milestone gave me a sense of control over the uncontrollable, transforming an uncertain future into a vision I could work toward daily.

Throughout my health journey, I've learned that progress isn't linear at all, it's shaped by how well we integrate the past, present, and future into every decision. There was a time when I felt trapped in reflection, reviewing past mistakes and wondering how I got here. Then I would shift into future anxiety, worrying about my prognosis and whether I was doing enough. The real breakthrough came when I realized that true change happens only in the present moment, on the Knife Edge of Time.

I began applying this concept practically:

- **Past:** I examined my old health patterns so as not to dwell on regret, but to identify what had truly worked for me and what hadn't.

- **Present:** I focused on taking decisive action each day, whether it was following a nutrition plan, engaging in meaningful movement, or embracing moments of rest without guilt.

- **Future:** Instead of fearing what was to come, I set small, realistic goals that built toward a larger vision of health and resilience.

This shift made all the difference. My past became a teacher, my future became a source of motivation, but the present became my power center. Every major breakthrough, whether in physical recovery, emotional resilience, or personal growth, happened when I embraced the present and committed to acting right now.

The Knife Edge Of Time

Time is universal, yet our experience of it is deeply personal. For Titans navigating the complexities of a diagnosis, time becomes more than just hours on a clock as it transforms into a resource that feels simultaneously abundant yet fleeting. It's measured in cycles of treatments, moments of waiting, and milestones of progress or setbacks.

By thinking about time as a continuously moving knife edge, with the edge being now, we redefine our relationship with time as a resource. Time is not a linear progression but a dynamic continuum of three dimensions:

- **The Past,** offering lessons.
- **The Future,** holding possibilities.
- **The Present,** the Knife Edge of Time, where action and transformation occur.

Instead of envisioning time as a precarious tightrope, picture it as a steady journey. The present second, the *knife edge of now,* is where clarity and motion intersect. It's the space where you take deliberate actions to navigate the lessons of the past and move toward the aspirations of the future. Behind you, the past provides insight, while ahead, the horizon stretches with possibilities. Your present focus determines the direction of your journey.

The Past: A Library of Lessons

Your past is a repository of wisdom. Think of it as a rearview mirror holding the experiences, challenges, and triumphs that have shaped you into who you are today. Revisiting it isn't about dwelling on regrets or reopening wounds. Instead, it's about understanding the Forces and Elements that brought you to this moment.

Mind: Your past holds memories of strategies and experiences that worked or failed. These moments teach you resilience and adaptability.

Body: Your body recalls its endurance, its scars, and its recoveries. Each one is a marker of your strength.

Soul: Your soul remembers moments of deep meaning, connection, and purpose that sustained you.

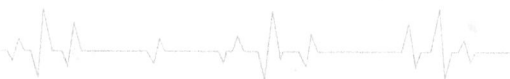

The Present: Where Action Exists

The present is the only place where action happens. It is the *Knife Edge of Time*, the moment where clarity and motion intersect. Picture yourself in the driver's seat of a car: the world outside may appear calm, yet every choice you make from steering and accelerating, to braking actively shapes your journey forward. This moment, while seemingly still, is the dynamic point of transformation.

Imagine standing on this edge: you cannot dwell on the road behind you, nor can you rush toward the horizon ahead. Your attention must remain on the now with most of your focus guiding the steady hands on the wheel that determines your direction. This metaphor captures the essence of the *Knife Edge of Time*:

- It is fleeting (this second right now), yet it is the only moment that exists.
- It is powerful because decisions made here shape everything that follows.

One of the most transformative lessons I learned was that every decision is made in the precise time stamped moment of your T0. Think of it this way, T-1 is the first second in the past, and behind it, all time previously. In the opposite direction is T+1 and all time past that into the future. Now, the second you are living and actually doing things being T0. In decoding terms, the past holds wisdom, the future holds goals, but the only moment that truly exists is now because the future starts just one second away.

Applying this concept changed the way I approached my health decisions:

- Instead of regretting past choices, I used them as reference points for smarter decisions.
- Instead of fearing the future, I took control of the present moment to shape it.
- Instead of feeling overwhelmed by long-term goals, I broke them into daily, actionable steps.

This shift in perspective allowed me to navigate my health challenges with clarity, confidence, and a renewed sense of purpose.

Dynamic Harmony Across Time

Embracing The Knife Edge Of Time means recognizing that the past, present, and future are not separate, they are interconnected. The lessons of the past inform your decisions today. Your actions in the present shape the future. And the aspirations of the future give meaning to the now.

This dynamic awareness shifts with your priorities: some days call for reflection, others demand action. The key is to remain adaptable, aligning your Mind, Body, and Soul with the rhythm of your lived experience.

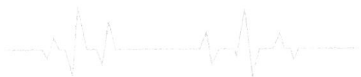

Aligning with The Knife Edge Of Time

The Knife Edge Of Time offers a new way to experience life's journey. It empowers you to harness the wisdom of the past, the aspirations of the future, and the clarity of the present. By embracing this framework, you can cultivate resilience, adapt to challenges, and create harmony across your Mind, Body, and Soul.

Recognizing time as a dynamic continuum is one thing, but how do you live it day to day, when your condition demands constant adaptation?

In the next chapter, we'll explore how to find sustainable balance within The Knife Edge Of Time in real life through systems, rituals, and habits that help you stay aligned, even when life pulls you in every direction.

Key Insight

The past is your teacher, the future is your vision, but the present is your power and the place of action where transformation begins.

Practical Reflections

Visit your past with curiosity, not judgment.

- What experiences, decisions, or patterns stand out?
- What lessons can you draw from them to guide your next steps?

Pause and take inventory of this present moment.

- What small, intentional action can you take right now to align your Mind, Body, and Soul?

The Future: A Horizon of Possibility

- **Mind:** Set intentions that reflect your values and priorities.
- **Body:** Create goals that align with your current health and energy levels.
- **Soul:** Envision a future filled with meaning and connection.

Imagine your future self, one year, five years, and a decade from now.
- What does that version of you look like?
- How does that version of you feel emotionally and mentally?
- What small steps can you take today to move closer to that vision?

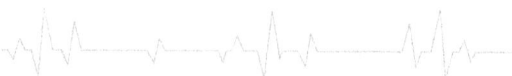

Fama's Sidebar:
Navigating the Knife Edge Of Time

Time isn't just about clocks and calendars, it's about choices. Going back to the car analogy, and you being behind the wheel. Behind you lies a road of lessons, ahead of you a horizon of possibilities, and beneath your hands the wheel of the present moment.

Each decision you make right now matters.

CHAPTER 10

Finding Balance within The Knife Edge Of Time

The concept of The Knife Edge Of Time came late in the philosophical development process. Yes, The Alignment concept worked ok without it, but every time I had a medical change of course for the worse, I found myself mentally trying to reconcile with the past again, almost trying to negotiate a better deal with 'the source' and promising to be a good boy if only I could rewire the past. If only I had a genie, everything would be good again. Of course, that was pointless.

It became even worse when I looked to my future, and how short it might be if this current dip kept going. With all these negative feedback loops I found myself returning to the slippery slope of defeat far too often, and as always Charlie was there on my shoulder like a cheerleader willing us towards the pending dome.

The first time I understood the Knife Edge of Time was on an actual highway west of Brisbane, Australia, driving to a site tender visit. I was halfway through another one of my medical dips, heart condition worsening even though I thought I was doing the right thing, uncertainty mounting, and the hum of the tyres beneath me, the hypnotic rhythm of the road, gave my thoughts space to wander.

In an effort of frustration, I started to consider what critical component was missing from the alignment process and how the gap in the theory allowed me to revert back to old thought patterns.

That's when it hit me: I was always either racing toward the future or staring into the past. What I was missing was the lane I was actually in, the present. The only lane where real movement happens.

I suddenly began deciphering the moment. There I was driving a car at high speed and yet I was personally (for all intent and purpose) stationary sitting in a driver's seat sipping a cool drink.

As I looked in the rearview mirror I could see the white lines rapidly retreating backwards where I had been with the past getting further and further away with every millisecond. As I looked forward again I could see the immediate future on the road ahead, but not

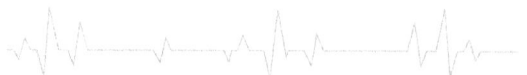

around the corner, not over the next rise, if I pulled over at the next service station, would I meet someone who would change my future. In fact, that exact event happened on the way back from the site (but that's another story). I had no idea what was going to happen in the future of my journey or that day.

After those two enlightening reflections I returned to inside the car as if it was the first time I had ever really explored what it means to be sitting stationary at speed and how, what I was doing now with my drink, with my hands on the wheel, and foot on the throttle, how this action right now had a direct impact on my future but no effect on my past. I laugh now but I tested my theory by roaming onto the audible bumps on the side of the lane just to prove what I did now, had an impact on the future.

I mean, this moment was a revelation to me and literally changed my view on life's time line completely.

This chapter is where the highway metaphor becomes more than just an analogy, it becomes a lens. Not just because it's poetic, but because it's personal.

Life, like a car speeding down a highway, moves relentlessly forward. For Titans navigating the challenges of a chronic diagnosis, time can feel both slow and overwhelming, a paradox of urgency and stillness. While the past may linger like a distant memory in the rearview mirror, the present demands constant decisions, and the future unfolds unpredictably with every mile.

The Origin of The Knife Edge Of Time

Driving in silence that day, after my revelation, I was mesmerised by the landscape gradually changing, not with sudden jumps, but through a series of small, continuous movements. That was it. Time wasn't just past-present-future like blocks on a calendar. It was motion in action. The past trailing behind like a dusty highway, the future stretching ahead, unknowable. But right here, where my hands gripped the wheel, that was the Knife Edge of Time. A place of clarity, of choice, of control. Of Action.

In this moment of discovery, the metaphor crystallized. Every Titan walks a similar road not knowing where the next turn leads, sometimes with fog ahead, sometimes on a steep incline. But the power lies in staying present behind the wheel. Every steering decision matters. Drifting off into the past or fixating too long on the horizon? That's how you miss an exit. Or worse, how you crash.

When my heart crash occurred, in those first few months of the heart disease diagnosis, I was forced to confront how precious and fragile time really was. But I drew strength from a fundamental truth: I had faced adversity before with prostate disease and have come out stronger. My experience with prostate cancer taught me that healing doesn't happen all at once, it's built on the foundation of daily actions and clarity of purpose.

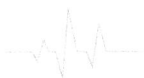

In those difficult days of cardiac recovery, I began viewing time not as an enemy but as a powerful ally with the future and the past of no immediate concern other than for reflection and planning. I created simple rituals to reconnect with what mattered:

- I reflected each morning on a single question: *What is one thing I can do today that my future self will thank me for?*

- I journaled moments of growth to prevent my mind from spiraling.

- I celebrated small wins such as deep breaths, restful nights, and heartfelt conversations.

I wasn't chasing perfection. I was practicing presence.

Navigating The Knife Edge Of Time

The Knife Edge Of Time isn't about controlling the clock, it's about shifting how you engage with time. It offers a flexible framework for realignment through three dimensions:

The Past: Your Rearview Mirror

Your past is rich with insight. Reflecting on previous struggles and breakthroughs provides a library of wisdom to draw from without dwelling in regret.

- Reflect on what has worked for you in the past and acknowledge the strength those moments required.

- Acknowledge the patterns or choices that have shaped your current path. Recognize which ones brought you strength and which ones may need to evolve and commit to navigating forward with intention.

- Commit to bringing those effective patterns forward into your present approach.

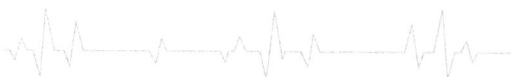

The Present: The Knife Edge of Time

This is your point of power. Here and now, you decide how to act. Every breath, every step, every thought has the potential to shift your trajectory.

- Identify a specific action you will take today to align your elements.

- Tune in to your Mind, Body, and Soul and decipher which one is asking for care or realignment today? Act with purpose in response to that call.

- Commit to this choice as a conscious step toward reclaiming your journey on the Knife Edge of Time.

The Future: A Horizon of Possibility

Your future is unwritten. It can feel uncertain, but it's also filled with hope and potential. By setting flexible goals, you give yourself something to move toward without becoming fixated.

- Like we did in the previous chapter, envision your life one year from now with an aligned dynamic harmony. Anchor that image in your heart and start treating it as your destination.

- Name one step you are ready to take today that supports your future alignment. Start small, but start now and don't look back.

Once you begin to navigate time with greater awareness, learning from the past, acting in the present, and shaping the future, you begin to see patterns of growth emerge. But growth doesn't happen automatically. It requires a mindset willing to adapt, learn, and persist through challenge. In the next chapter, we'll explore how to embrace that mindset, so you can move forward with clarity and strength, even when the road ahead feels uncertain.

Key Insight

You don't control time but you can choose how you move through it. Aligning your decisions with The Knife Edge Of Time allows your past to teach you, your present to empower you, and your future to inspire you.

Practical Reflections

Use your Alignment Workbook to explore the following:

- **Past:** Reclaim a moment of strength or learning from your past and let it guide your next decision. Let it remind you that progress has already been made, and that wisdom is already yours to build from.

- **Present:** Choose one small, intentional action that aligns your Mind, Body, or Soul today. Commit to it as a declaration that you're living fully on the Knife Edge of Time.

- **Future:** Anchor a powerful vision of who you are becoming. Let that image inspire a step today that brings it closer to the reality that can be your tomorrow.

Fama's Sidebar
When Roads Don't Exist

When the highway doesn't lead where you need to go, it's time to cut your own path. This isn't just a detour, it's a bold act of creating the life you deserve.

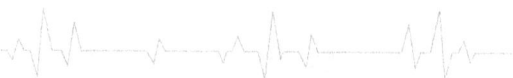

Unlock Action Now With The Alignment Workbook

Reading *Decode Your Diagnosis* is a powerful step but information alone doesn't change a life. What changes a life is action. And for Titans, whether you are living with a diagnosis, caring for someone you love, or supporting patients in a clinical role, action can feel overwhelming without the right tools.

That's why *The Alignment Workbook* exists. It's not another journal to collect dust on your nightstand. It's a structured, practical guide designed to help you apply the ideas you've just read. Inside, you'll find simple check-ins, clear exercises, and small alignment actions that give you momentum, clarity, and hope.

For the patient, this workbook helps you turn theory into daily progress. For the carer, it creates shared language and practices to walk alongside the one you love. And for the clinician, it offers a way to integrate the Decode Your Diagnosis framework into conversations and support beyond the clinic walls.

This is your action tool. A bridge from theory to practice. A way to move from simply *understanding* your diagnosis to actively decoding it, one step at a time.

Visit the Decode Your Diagnosis website to grab your copy now from:

decodeyourdiagnosis.com

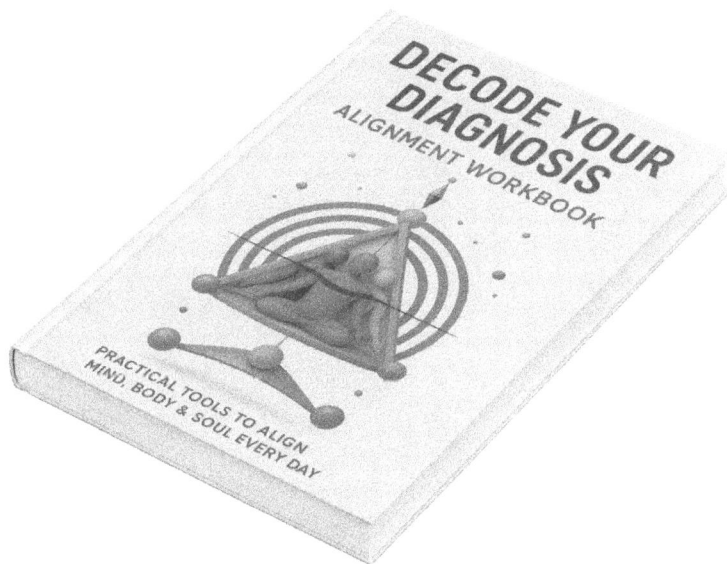

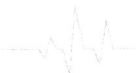

CHAPTER 11

Embracing a Growth Mindset

Embodying resilience during a medical setback like my heart crash of 2024, was one of the most defining moments of my health journey.

At the time, I didn't have a formal framework to follow, but I was journaling daily, trying to make sense of my rapid decline. In doing so, I realized that I needed a structured approach to navigate this crisis. That realization became the seed for what would eventually become the decision models I rely on today.

I was in medical freefall. If I didn't take immediate action, I knew I would be facing a life-threatening event within a matter of weeks.

To regain control, I developed a crude version of a decision tree, mapping out all potential causes and solutions:

- Was my stress load too high?
- Was I overexerting myself physically?
- Were my medications interacting poorly?

By going through this process, I identified root causes, engaged my psychologist to help with mental and emotional load, and made critical adjustments to my treatment plan. The result? A complete stabilization within eight weeks and return to work.

This experience reinforced the power of structured decision-making in managing chronic illness.

Self-compassion has been a constant struggle for me, and as a Titan, managing the comorbidity of heart disease and prostate disease, that struggle became even more apparent. The turning point came during a therapy session when I caught myself berating my body for being "weaker" than it used to be. My psychologist gently interrupted and asked, "Would you speak to a friend that way?" That moment landed hard. It was the first time I saw how cruel my internal dialogue had become. From then on, I began practicing moments of self-kindness, not perfectly, but with increasing awareness that compassion isn't a luxury, it's a necessity.

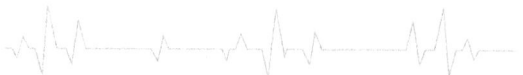

In the summer of 2024, we decided to sell our home of 29 years. Maintaining acreage wasn't feasible long-term, and we didn't want to wait until my heart condition worsened to make a move.

Despite promising my wife I wouldn't overexert myself, guilt got the better of me. One weekend, I jumped in to help clear under the house and pushed myself like nothing had changed. By 11am, I felt spaced out, was completely drained and looked ghostly white. My wife intervened, sending me inside to recover and banishing me from further physical activity relating to the house cleanup.

It took hours of full mental and physical rest and a nap before I felt remotely normal again.

That moment was a turning point. I realized that my own expectations of myself were unrealistic, I was still measuring my capabilities by my pre-diagnosis standards. That needed to change.

I learned that resilience is not just about pushing forward, it's about knowing when to stop. Adjusting my mindset around self-compassion and introducing meditation to provide moments of mental rest and reflection became critical assistants for managing the condition effectively.

In yet another example when I was diagnosed with prostate disease, I knew surgery was necessary and like many men diagnosed with this condition, the fear of losing my masculinity clouded my decision-making process. I am informed that women undergo similar concerns when it comes to breast cancer and femininity.

In my case, I was yet to consider the alternatives.

At 50 years old, the thought of incontinence and erectile dysfunction felt devastating. Despite knowing I needed intervention, I was yet to understand what it would mean for my identity.

What shifted my perspective?

- Pelvic floor physiotherapy and realizing that incontinence wasn't a guaranteed outcome if I took proactive steps.
- Conversations with a prostate cancer nurse who walked me through the realities of surgery and recovery.
- Recognizing that survival mattered more than outdated societal perceptions.

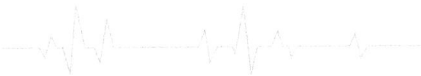

Once I made peace with my decision, I realized that true resilience means embracing change, even when it challenges our deeply held beliefs. It reminded me of the bold simplicity of a Katherine Hamnett t-shirt, the kind Wham! made famous in the '80s; *CHOOSE LIFE.*

Unapologetic, direct, and refusing to be ignored. Just like the shirt's defiant message, this realization challenged me to redefine strength, not as control or perfection, but as the willingness to adapt, accept, and choose life on new terms.

The Core Elements of a Growth Mindset

Resilience Through Setbacks

Life with a diagnosis is rarely linear. A growth mindset helps you see setbacks not as failures but as stepping stones. Titans can navigate setbacks by:

- Identifying the Internal Force (e.g., fear, frustration) and External Force (e.g., isolation, conflicting advice) creating imbalance.
- Focusing attention on the affected Element.
- Finding small, meaningful steps to restore Dynamic Harmony and keep moving forward.

Example: A Titan faces a fitness setback after an injury. By identifying frustration (Internal) and physical limitations (External), they focus on Body, selecting restorative actions like stretching or mindfulness until recovery.

The Role of Self-Compassion

A growth mindset thrives on self-compassion, the practice of treating yourself with kindness. Self-compassion can be practiced intentionally by aligning decisions with Dynamic Harmony. For example:

- **Mind:** Reflective journaling to process self-doubt.
- **Body:** Prioritizing rest during periods of fatigue.
- **Soul:** Engaging in gratitude practices to reconnect with purpose.

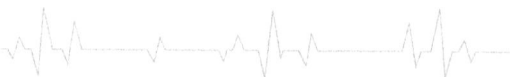

The 'Yet' Perspective

When faced with a chronic diagnosis, it's easy to feel trapped by limitations and the overwhelming weight of what lies ahead. But what if every challenge, every setback, every struggle could be reframed as an opportunity for growth? Enter the power of "yet."

The word "yet" transforms defeat into possibility. It turns "I can't do this" into "I can't do this yet." This simple shift in perspective forms the foundation of a growth mindset, a way of thinking that embraces challenges, values learning, and sees potential in every situation.

One of the simplest yet most profound tools in cultivating a growth mindset is adding the word "yet" to your inner dialogue.

- "I can't feel balanced" becomes "I can't feel balanced yet."

- "I don't know how to move forward" becomes "I don't know how to move forward yet."

This perspective transforms "yet" into tangible progress.

Extending Growth Past Treatment

After treatment we enter into what is called the Survivorship phase, and it is about maintaining resilience and sustaining healthy habits. Titans can strengthen their focus by making small adjustments to daily routines while keeping long-term goals in view.

Example: A Titan re-prioritizes Body after a period of physical complacency, choosing small steps like walking or meal prepping to rebuild momentum.

Reinvention

The Ultimate Expression of Growth

Reinvention moves beyond stability into creativity and contribution. The growth mindset shines here, enabling Titans to set new goals and align their decodingwith purpose.

Example: A Titan in Reinvention explores Soul-focused actions, such as starting a passion project or mentoring others.

Practical Integration

Daily Practices to Cultivate a Growth Mindset

Reframing Challenges

Turn setbacks into growth opportunities:

- Identify forces causing imbalance
- Focus on the affected Element.
- Select a Dynamic Harmony action and reflect on its impact.

Tracking Small Wins

Document daily progress, no matter how small. Celebrate victories aligned with your Trinity.

Visioning for Reinvention

Imagine what life could look like in Reinvention. Reinvention tends to happen after we have decoded the diagnosis and after any clinical intervention. It's when we can start to reflect on who we were before the condition and who we would like to reinvent ourselves to become in the future. What passions or goals have you put on hold? Break these aspirations into achievable steps.

Growth begins with belief, but it deepens with awareness. In order to move forward, you must first understand where you are now and where, or more importantly who you'd like to be in the future.. In the next chapter, we'll take a closer look at how awareness and self-compassion work hand in hand to help you build the emotional and mental resilience needed to decode your diagnosis and stay aligned with your deeper purpose.

Key Insight

A growth mindset isn't about relentless positivity, it's about courageous adaptability. Titans grow not by denying setbacks, but by reframing them into progress, one intentional step at a time.

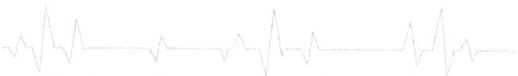

Practical Reflections

Before moving on to the next chapter let's remember that a growth mindset isn't a destination, it's a way of navigating life. By embracing the power of "yet," practicing self-compassion, and staying aligned, you can transform challenges into opportunities for growth and resilience.

Your diagnosis doesn't define you, how you choose to respond does.

- Think of a current doubt related to your diagnosis and transform it into a "yet" expression.
- Take your "yet" expression and consider some action you can apply to address your yet expression now or in the near future.
- Write down what a growth mindset looks like for your diagnosis.

Fama's Sidebar
Harnessing the Power of Yet

The word 'yet' is small but mighty. It's a reminder that growth is always possible, even when the path feels hard. When you face setbacks, pause and ask yourself: What can I learn from this? How does this challenge make me stronger? Every step forward, no matter how small, is a victory. Remember, resilience isn't about how fast you grow, it's about staying committed to the journey. You've got this.

CHAPTER 12

Building Awareness and Self-Compassion

Awareness is the starting point for transformation. When you build awareness, you open a window to understanding your thoughts, emotions, and behaviors. It's through this understanding that you begin to uncover your strengths and address your challenges, laying the groundwork for growth.

But awareness is only part of the equation. It must be paired with self-compassion which, in it's simplest form, is the practice of treating yourself with kindness, patience, and understanding, especially during difficult times. This balance between awareness and compassion creates a powerful synergy, enabling you to navigate life's challenges with resilience.

When I was first diagnosed with prostate disease, I believed that simply following medical advice was enough. I relied solely on my doctors and ignored my own intuition. But in reality, I wasn't self-aware at all because I was disconnected from what was happening to my body and what having cancer really meant. I assumed that if I followed instructions, everything would be fine.

It wasn't until my heart disease diagnosis that my wife confronted me about my lack of awareness. She had noticed the signs long before I had: the fatigue, the subtle shifts in my energy, the moments of irritability I had brushed off. She had tried to bring it up, but I dismissed her concerns as over-worrying.

That moment was a wake-up call. I realized that I needed to take an active role in understanding my health. With my wife's help, I started tracking my symptoms, energy levels, and lifestyle patterns. Over time, I identified clear links between my daily habits and my wellbeing. I wasn't just a patient, I was finally becoming an engaged participant in my own health. This shift in perspective gave me confidence and control, allowing me to make informed decisions rather than reactive ones.

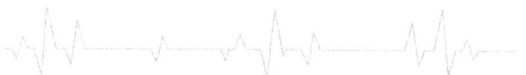

Awareness is an important tool for navigating The Alignment Pathway, helping to identify patterns and choose intentional actions for alignment. It's not about judgment but observation. The goal is to see life as it is, not as we wish it to be, and to use that understanding as a foundation for intentional change.

Looking back, my body had been signaling distress long before I was diagnosed with heart disease. The problem was, I wasn't paying attention.

- **Frequent fatigue became "just being busy"**
- **Irritability was blamed on work stress.**
- **High stress levels were dismissed as part of my career.**

Only after my heart disease diagnosis did I connect these dots. Had I recognized the warning signs earlier, I could have intervened sooner. This realization reinforced the importance of listening to my body, not just medical test results.

One of the hardest lessons I had to learn was how to be kind to myself. When the condition worsened, I fell into a pattern of blaming myself for past decisions, the poor diet, the constant stress and if I'm honest with myself, the lack of exercise. The guilt was overwhelming.

It wasn't until I worked with my psychologist that I realized this mindset was counterproductive. Instead of punishing myself for the past, I needed to focus on the present and future. I reframed setbacks as learning opportunities, giving myself the grace to adjust without self-judgment.

For a long time during the prostate cancer treatment , I saw my chronic illness as something happening to me like a cruel twist of fate. It felt like I had boarded a train with no control over its destination, moving forward whether I was ready or not.

But reframing my story changed so many aspects. Instead of being a passenger, I decided to take the wheel. Like all best trips of randomness I let go of the plan and discovered new paths, I began navigating my own health my way, adapting as I went along.

Instead of seeing myself as a victim of prostate disease or cancer, I began seeing myself as a Titan on a journey. This wasn't about "fighting" my diagnosis, it was about embracing resilience, adapting to detours, and choosing a pathway that empowered me.

This mindset shift helped me stay motivated, even on difficult days. I wasn't powerless. I had a say in my future. And just like in travel, the key was not resisting change but learning to navigate it with confidence.

The Power of Awareness

Awareness and self-compassion are not standalone practices, they are essential tools for navigating your health journey. Together, they provide the clarity and courage to embrace a fresh perspective to reframe your diagnosis as an opportunity. This is not about denying its challenges but seeing it as a catalyst for growth, change, and self-discovery. An empowered diagnosis acknowledges the complexity of your situation while equipping you with the tools to face it head-on.

Awareness helps you understand the Forces and Elements at play in your life. It reveals patterns in your thoughts, behaviors, and environment that influence your health and well-being. With awareness, you can identify the habits and beliefs that either support or hinder your journey.

Self-Compassion: Your Ally in the Journey

Self-compassion is the practice of offering yourself the same kindness and understanding you would offer a dear friend. It's especially important when you're navigating the emotional landscape of a diagnosis.

A lack of self-compassion can lead to harsh self-criticism, guilt, or feelings of inadequacy, all of which drain your energy and hinder progress. In contrast, self-compassion provides a safe space to process your emotions, learn from your experiences, and move forward with resilience.

Kristin Neff, a leading researcher on self-compassion, outlines three core components of this practice:

- **Self-kindness:** Treating yourself with warmth and understanding instead of harsh criticism.
- **Common humanity:** Recognizing that struggles are part of the shared human experience.
- **Mindfulness:** Observing your thoughts and feelings without becoming overwhelmed by them.

When self-compassion becomes a daily practice, it helps restore balance across the decoding coal face, enabling the Mind, Body, and Soul to realign after setbacks.

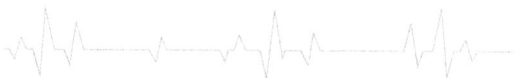

Empowered Diagnosis: A New Perspective

An empowered diagnosis shifts the narrative. Instead of seeing your diagnosis as an end, you see it as a beginning. It's an opportunity to:

• Build a deeper understanding of your Mind, Body, and Soul.
• Make intentional choices that align with your values.
• Develop resilience and strength through adversity.

An empowered diagnosis integrates the decoding philosophy, helping you navigate Forces with resilience and align with your purpose. It's not about minimizing the reality of your condition but about reclaiming agency over your life and taking steps to create a meaningful future.

Steps to Build Awareness and Self-Compassion

Observe Your Inner Dialogue

• Pay attention to the way you talk to yourself. Is your inner voice kind and supportive, or critical and harsh?
• Write down recurring thoughts and reflect on how they shape your emotions and actions.

Practice Mindful Observation

• Set aside a few minutes each day to observe your thoughts, feelings, and bodily sensations without judgment.
• This practice helps you build awareness and strengthens your connection to the present moment.

Write a Self-Compassion Letter

• Imagine a dear friend is facing the same challenges you are. Write them a letter offering support, encouragement, and understanding.
• Then, read the letter back to yourself, recognizing that you deserve the same compassion.

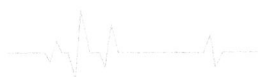

Reframe Negative Beliefs

- Identify one negative belief you hold about your diagnosis.
- Challenge its validity and reflect on how this belief impacts your Mind, Body, and Soul.
- Reframe it in a way that strengthens alignment. For example, "I'm too weak to handle this" can become "I have faced challenges before, and I am capable of growing through this one."

Each of these practices builds the foundation for greater clarity, alignment, and resilience, helping you make decisions that reflect both awareness and compassion.

Awareness opens the door, but it's compassion that allows you to walk through it. Now that you've begun listening more deeply to your thoughts, emotions, and body, the next step is learning how to meet what you find with kindness. In the next chapter, we'll explore how to cultivate self-compassion, not as a soft ideal, but as a powerful force for healing and resilience.

Key Insight

Self-awareness and self-compassion don't remove life's challenges, but they do have the potential to change how you face them. Together, they help you move from reaction to intention, and from limitation to possibility.

Practical Reflection

A Commitment to Self-Kindness

Reflect on the role of your internal support, of self-compassion in your journey.

Imagine your future self looking back on this moment. What would they thank you for?

There are some practical questions as well and here they are.

- What beliefs about your diagnosis are influencing your Mind, Body, and Soul?
- Are they empowering or limiting each element?
- How do your daily habits affect your Mind, Body, and Soul?
- What external Forces are shaping your journey, positively or negatively?

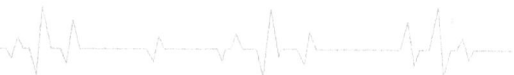

Fama's Sidebar
Building Awareness with Your Navigator

Today, let's take a step toward deeper awareness. When you reflect on your journey, remember that every thought and feeling is a clue or a piece of the puzzle that makes up your story. Together, we can use these clues to chart a path forward. Start by asking yourself: What am I feeling right now, and why? Awareness is the first step toward empowerment.

CHAPTER 13

The Power of
Self-Compassion

Imagine this: You've just had a setback. Maybe your symptoms flare up unexpectedly. The inner critic swoops in: "Why didn't I do more?" But what if you paused, took a breath, and instead said: "This is tough, but I'm doing the best I can."

That's self-compassion. It's about learning to treat yourself with the same understanding and patience you would extend to a friend. It's not about ignoring mistakes or challenges; it's about responding to them in a way that promotes resilience and growth. For Titans, self-compassion can become a steady companion, helping you navigate life's ups and downs with grace.

What Does Self-Compassion Look Like?

Self-compassion is a skill that you can develop, and it starts with small, intentional acts of kindness toward yourself. Let's break it down:

- **Self-Kindness:** Imagine speaking to yourself like you would to someone you deeply care about. Instead of saying, "I can't believe I failed again," you might say, "I gave it my best shot, and that was enough."
- **Common Humanity:** Think back to a time when you struggled and felt alone. Now remind yourself that everyone faces challenges. You're not broken; you're human, and that's a shared experience.
- **Mindfulness:** Picture a river flowing calmly. Each thought and emotion is a leaf floating by. Mindfulness is about observing those leaves without clinging to them or pushing them away. You simply watch them drift.

These principles weave together to create a mindset that nurtures growth and helps Titans maintain alignment across Mind, Body, and Soul.

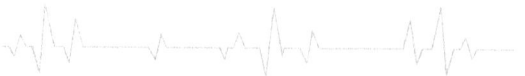

Why Does Self-Compassion Matter?

Let's imagine two Titans. One faces a setback and berates themselves, spiraling into frustration and self-doubt. The other takes a moment to breathe and reminds themselves that setbacks are opportunities to learn. Which Titan do you think will move forward with more clarity and resilience?

Self-compassion doesn't erase challenges, but it changes how you face them. It can:

- **Boost Resilience:** Helping you bounce back from difficulties faster.
- **Calm Your Inner Critic:** Quieting that harsh voice in your head that says you're not enough.
- **Strengthen Your Trinity:** Aligning your Mind, Body, and Soul through acts of kindness.

Barriers to Self-Compassion

It's not always easy to be kind to yourself. You might think, "Isn't self-compassion just an excuse to slack off?" Or, "If I'm too soft on myself, won't I lose my drive?" These are common misconceptions. Self-compassion isn't about letting yourself off the hook. It's about treating your effort with fairness and choosing to move forward with intention.

Other barriers might include:

- **Perfectionism:** Believing you must get everything right to be worthy of compassion.

  At the time of my prostate disease diagnosis, I was a perfectionist. I wanted to maintain control, even when control was no longer an option. My inner critic bombarded me with relentless self-doubt: "How could this happen to me? Why didn't I prevent myself from getting cancer?"

  The cycle was endless. I couldn't switch it off. That was, until I read *Solve for Happy* by Mo Gawdat. In his book, he suggested naming your inner critic to create distance from its negativity. Once I gave my inner critic a name, I could finally talk to him like a noisy neighbour: "Thanks, Charlie. I've heard you but I am focusing on the next step for now."

  This small shift in perspective helped me regain control, not over my diagnosis, but over my response to it. Self-compassion wasn't about eliminating fears; it was about learning to live with them in a healthier way.

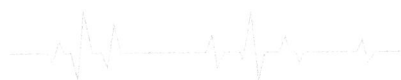

- **Cultural Norms:** Growing up in environments that equate toughness with strength.

Healing after a major medical event, like my heart crash in 2024, required more than just physical recovery, it required emotional healing, too.

When I saw my heart health drop from 60% to 42% in a matter of weeks, I was overwhelmed with guilt. How had I let it get this bad? Wasn't I doing everything right? I was so caught up in blaming myself that I failed to see the larger picture.

It wasn't until I took a step back and worked with my mental health professional that I realized something crucial: The heart crash wasn't a failure. It was a signal. My body was communicating an imbalance in the heart disease, and it was up to me to listen and adjust.

By shifting my perspective from self-blame to self-awareness, I was able to focus on solutions rather than regrets. I identified stress as a key factor, made lifestyle changes, and within months, my heart health had rebounded beyond where it had started. Self-compassion was not just a comfort, it was a necessary tool for recovery.

- **Fear of Vulnerability:** Worrying that being kind to yourself is a sign of weakness.

For years, I resisted vulnerability. I wanted to appear strong, capable, in control. But chronic illness doesn't care about appearances.

One of the greatest lessons I've learned is that embracing vulnerability doesn't mean giving up, it means accepting where I am and taking action from that place of honesty. During the AcuGraph organ function test the results were clear: My health had improved more in the last year, since embracing a decoding mindset, than it had for a long time.

Why? Because I stopped striving for perfection and started focusing on alignment. Instead of trying to force my body into an ideal state, I learned to work with it.

By prioritizing balance over unattainable perfection, I was achieving measurable progress. Instead of pretending I had everything under control, I sought support and allowed myself to grow.

Recognizing these barriers IS the first step to breaking through them.

Cultivating self-compassion is not a solitary journey. As you learn to treat yourself with kindness, it naturally opens space for deeper connection with others. In the next chapter, we explore how surrounding yourself with the right people and support structures can multiply your resilience and help carry the weight of your diagnosis together.

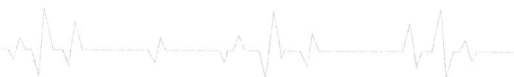

Key Insight

Self-compassion is not a sign of weakness, it's a powerful act of strength. When you meet yourself with kindness, you create the emotional foundation for real, lasting growth.

Practical Reflections

This chapter is short but its concept is often overlooked by us all because it seems weird to offer ourselves self-compassion. As a gesture of encouragement I am going to ask you to do two things in this practical reflection. First, do something right now as an affirmation in the form of a call-to-action and then follow through with the regular exercises in the Awareness Workbook.

Call-to-Action

Take a moment today to reflect on how you speak to yourself. Practice self-compassion in a small way whether it's by reframing a self-critical thought or taking a deep breath when challenges arise. You are always welcome over in the Decode your Diagnosis Substack publication to share your experiences.

Your Questions

- When was the last time you were hard on yourself?
- How did it affect your energy or outlook?
- What would it look like to meet that moment again with compassion instead of criticism?
- What's one kind thing you can say to yourself today to support your Alignment?

Fama's Sidebar

Self-compassion isn't about ignoring mistakes or challenges; it's about meeting them with kindness. What's one kind thing you can say to yourself today? Small acts of self-compassion lead to big changes over time. Remember, you're doing the best you can.

CHAPTER 14

Finding Your Support Network

Facing a chronic diagnosis like cancer or prostate disease, can feel isolating. The instinct to bear the weight alone is common, but the truth is no one should navigate their healing journey in isolation. A resilient support network isn't just a resource; it's an integral part of the journey. It acts as a safety net during setbacks, access to knowledgeable guides when the path becomes unclear, and a source of encouragement when challenges feel insurmountable.

The moment of diagnosis is a particularly difficult time, and I must admit it was overwhelming when I was told I was at the extreme end of heart disease and considered incurable.

It's during these moments that we need the solace of a true confidant. In my case, I have been fortunate to share a marriage of over thirty years, and my wife has been my strongest ally and closest confidant.

She knew exactly how this diagnosis would affect me. With gentle, well-timed prompting, she gave me the space to process my emotions while also offering reassurances like, *"You're not alone in this."* As the reality of the condition settled in, her consistent support reminded me of the importance of self-compassion.

At times, her observations about my mental state were instrumental in nudging me toward taking the next steps in my care. I didn't always feel like embracing it, without her encouragement though, my journey through recovery would have been harder, slower, and less effective.

Not all support networks are created equal. The strongest ones offer more than companionship, they reflect your values, provide emotional and practical help, and align with your personal goals.

Before building the ideal support network, it's important to assess where we are. What relationships and resources do we currently rely on, and how well do they serve our needs?

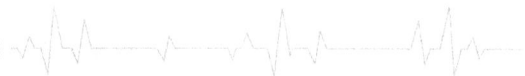

Choosing the right professional network for my decoding Team was critical to achieving the best possible outcome. Dealing with heart disease required assembling a broad, interdisciplinary team spanning modern medicine, Traditional Chinese Medicine, Ayurvedic treatment, and naturopathy.

One of the most essential figures in my decoding team is my naturopath. I refer to her as my *Functional Integration* Coach because she plays a pivotal role in evaluating the combined impact of all my treatments. She ensures that:

- There are no overlapping medications or contraindications between my prescribed treatments.
- My diet, supplements, and herbal regimens complement my medical treatments rather than conflict with them.
- I maintain a holistic approach to managing the condition rather than relying on fragmented solutions.

Her careful evaluations have saved me from potential negative interactions and helped optimize my treatment plan. Having a trusted expert to oversee the broader integration of treatments has been one of my biggest assets in managing the condition.

One of the hardest parts of chronic illness is that you can't talk about it with just anyone. There are stigmas associated with certain conditions, and sometimes, even well-meaning friends and family members struggle to relate. The result? A sense of alienation, even among those who care.

I quickly learned that to thrive, I needed to find people who truly understood my experience. That's why I created *The Titans Arena*, an online community where Titans can openly share their struggles, victories, and strategies for resilience.

For those who prefer in-person connection, local support groups, fitness communities, and wellness circles can also be invaluable. I've found incredible support within my yoga community, where I've had deep and meaningful conversations with fellow Titans navigating their own health challenges.

Wherever you find your community, make sure it fosters growth, empowerment, and mutual support.

The Power of a Support Network

In the Decode Your Diagnosis framework, the Mind, Body, and Soul must remain in harmony and so must your support network. Each relationship and resource should amplify your resilience, mirroring the balance you strive for within. Building this system takes intentionality and courage, but the rewards are profound: a network that uplifts you, helps you navigate challenges, and celebrates your progress.

What Makes a Support Network Effective?

Key Characteristics of Effective Support:

- **Trust:** You feel safe sharing your fears, hopes, and needs.
- **Understanding:** Empathy and nonjudgmental listening create connection.
- **Expertise:** Professional guidance, from medical advice to coaching, grounds your decisions in knowledge.
- **Shared Purpose:** Supporters align with your values and goals, respecting your unique path.

Support comes in many forms:

- **Emotional Support:** Comfort, validation, and a listening ear.
- **Practical Support:** Assistance with daily tasks or planning.
- **Informational Support:** Access to knowledge, expertise, and resources.

A balanced support network integrates all three types, creating a robust foundation for your journey.

Building your Aligned Support Network

Your support network should mirror the harmony you seek within yourself. Let's explore how to align your network with the three pillars of decoding:

Mind: Mental Clarity and Resilience

- Seek out mentors, therapists, or trusted friends who encourage growth and help you process emotions constructively.
- Tools like mindfulness coaching or Titan groups can foster clarity.

Example: A friend who actively listens without judgment can ease the burden of doubt and provide perspective.

Body: Physical Health and Vitality

- Build a team of reliable medical professionals, nutritionists, or fitness coaches.
- Find accountability partners who motivate you to stay consistent with health goals.

Example: A workout partner or nutritionist can help you maintain energy and strength, even on tough days.

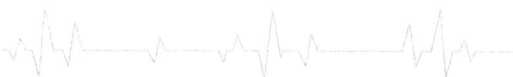

Soul: Meaning and Connection

- Surround yourself with people who inspire and uplift you, whether through shared values, spirituality, or creative passions.
- Look for communities or mentors aligned with your purpose.

Example: A creative group or spiritual advisor can reignite your sense of joy and fulfillment.

Fear of vulnerability, cultural expectations, and past disappointments can make building a support network challenging. Recognizing and addressing these barriers is essential to creating meaningful connections.

Strategies for Overcoming Barriers

- **Start Small:** Begin with one trusted person before expanding your network.
- **Seek Professional Guidance:** Therapists or coaches can help you navigate trust issues or cultural expectations.
- **Be Intentional:** Prioritize quality over quantity; deep, meaningful relationships matter more than a large network.

Building a community of like-minded Titans is vital for staying connected and maintaining resilience.

Practical Tools and Strategies

Creating and maintaining a support network requires intentional effort. These tools can help:

Creating A Support Network Map

There is an exercise at the end of the chapter to help you with this as a task. For now however;

- Visualize your current network.
- Include activity like exercise
- Highlight areas of strength and identify gaps needing attention.

Conduct A Connection Audit

- Evaluate the quality of each relationship. Ask yourself:
  - Does this person uplift or drain me?
  - Do they align with my values and goals?

Alignment Awareness

• Reflect on how new connections support the alignment of your Mind, Body, or Soul:
    - Which Element does this person help strengthen?
    - How does their presence impact your alignment and well-being?

The Path Forward

Your support network is a living, evolving entity, just like your Dynamic Harmony. It bridges the gap between your internal Elements and external Forces, amplifying your ability to adapt and thrive. Relationships that once felt distant may become closer, while new connections may emerge as pivotal allies along your journey.

As you move forward, remember: a strong support network isn't just a resource, it's a source of transformation. Let it uplift you, guide you, and remind you that even in the hardest moments, you are never alone.

Quick Tips:

• Starting Conversations: Unsure how to begin? Try, *"I've been focusing on ways to take better care of myself and would value your perspective."*

• Seeking Professional Allies: Research online or ask for recommendations from trusted sources. Take the time to find someone who aligns with your needs.

• Creating a Ripple Effect: Building your resilience inspires those around you to grow as well. Your network is more than just a support mechanism, it's a community of shared strength.

In the next chapter, we'll explore how strengthening your Alignment Fitness can reinforce the resilience you've been building so your support network becomes not just a safety net, but a springboard.

Key Insight

A strong support network doesn't just hold you up, it helps you rise. The people you surround yourself with can either drain your energy or deepen your alignment. Choose connection with intention.

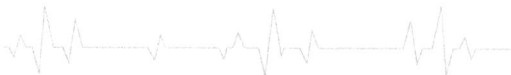

Exercise: Mapping Your Support Network

1. **List Your Network:** Write down the names of people you turn to for support, advice, or comfort.

2. **Categorize by decodingElement:**
   • Mind: Who helps you process emotions or gain clarity?
   • Body: Who supports your physical health or daily tasks?
   • Soul: Who nurtures your sense of purpose and connection?

3. **Evaluate Balance:**
   • Which categories feel strong?
   • Which ones need more attention?

This exercise reveals gaps and highlights opportunities to expand or strengthen your network.

Practical Reflections

- Who in your life helps you feel seen, heard, and understood without judgment or fixing?
- Which of your current relationships feel unbalanced or depleting?
- What boundaries might help?
- Which decoding Element (Mind, Body, or Soul) is least supported by your current network?
- What's one intentional step you can take this week to strengthen or expand your support system?

Fama's Sidebar
Building Your Network with Confidence

Building relationships isn't about perfection, it's about connection. Start small. Be intentional. Use your own judgement and reflection to guide you in choosing the right people and resources. Remember, every strong network begins with one meaningful conversation.

CHAPTER 15

Developing Alignment Fitness

What is Alignment Fitness?

Alignment Fitness is not about achieving perfection in one area of life but moreover about fostering balance and resilience across the interconnected Elements of the Mind, Body, and Soul. Unlike traditional views of fitness that focus solely on physical health, Alignment Fitness encompasses emotional clarity, physical vitality, and spiritual alignment.

For Titans navigating life with a chronic diagnosis, developing Alignment Fitness can feel overwhelming. But with the right mindset, professional guidance, and intentional practice, you can create a foundation of strength and adaptability that empowers you through every phase of your Pathway.

Finding Alignment Fitness can seem impossible at the moment of diagnosis because the first casulty is mental clarity. Rebuilding mental clarity requires support, and if your level of stress is as deep as mine was at the beginning of my heart disease diagnosis, your support needs to be professional.

During the first three months of my heart disease diagnosis, I sat on it, taking heed of my GP and cardiologist but doing little more. At the time, my career and balancing my new CEO role with family life were my priorities. Research shows that employees experiencing chronic work-related stress are at a significantly increased risk of coronary events. I was incurable, so I did nothing, stunned into inaction.

Physically, I was healthy, I had worked so hard to achieve that after my prostate disease journey, but mentally and spiritually, I was a mess. My wife saw it first, and my daughters noticed it too. They suggested professional help, and I reluctantly agreed.

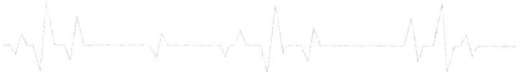

It turned out that internalized stress was damaging my physical health. Working with my psychologist, we peeled back years of suppressed stress. I could see the impact on my smart watch and my heart health, which had been steadily declining, leveled off as my mental clarity improved. Stress management wasn't optional, it was critical.

Physical setbacks can derail progress, but resilience means recalibrating rather than giving up.

When I liquidated our family business of 65 years, I thought that was rock bottom until I was diagnosed with prostate cancer a month later.

At the time, I was in a deep depression. My mental resilience was gone, and physically, I was in terrible shape still drinking alcohol, overweight, and neglecting my health entirely.

Prostate cancer saved my life.

The moment I committed to fighting cancer, physically I changed a lot:

- Quit drinking alcohol
- Started daily exercise
- Began tracking my health metrics

These small steps laid the foundation for my future recovery, proving that even in the darkest moments, reclaiming vitality is possible.

Fitness isn't just about physical health, it's about mental and spiritual endurance.

At the peak of my professional career, I was at my lowest point spiritually. The pressure of maintaining my leadership role, my family, and my health left me feeling disconnected and empty.

I redefined fitness by expanding it beyond just the body to an aligned perspective incorporating:

- **Mind:** Daily mental clarity exercises and stress journaling
- **Body:** Gentle, restorative movements rather than high-impact training
- **Soul:** Mindfulness practices, heartfulness meditation, and reconnecting with my creative side

Another shift happened when I discovered Kanha Shanti Vanam, a spiritual retreat that reintroduced me to the power of stillness, meditation, and a deeper connection to self. Immersing myself in that environment allowed me to recalibrate in a way that no amount of physical training ever could.

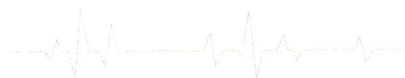

This functional fitness approach transformed my overall wellbeing, proving that fitness is about far more than just movement.

Yet another unexpected turning point came when I was undergoing prostate cancer treatment and stumbled upon The Core by Aki Hintsa. His model for high-performance wellbeing in the world of Formula 1 drivers completely reframed how I viewed alignment. As a motorsport enthusiast, I was captivated by how drivers didn't just train physically but they also lived intentionally, refining every aspect of life to sustain performance under pressure. Around the same time, I was reading The Barefoot Investor by Scott Pape, rethinking our financial future after the family business closed.

These books couldn't have been more different. One focused on elite physical and psychological conditioning, the other on practical financial stability, but both delivered a single, powerful message: *sustainable progress comes from clear values, simple systems, and long-term focus.*

I applied Hintsa's approach to my own health: analyzing internal and external Forces, building daily habits from my identity outward, and recalibrating whenever I veered off course. With Pape's method, I created space in my financial life, which reduced stress and freed energy to invest in Soul Fitness through creativity, connection, and stillness.

This pairing taught me that resilience isn't just surviving, it's structuring your life so you thrive under pressure. The lessons I learned here became part of my daily rhythm, embedding Alignment Fitness not just as a goal, but as a way of being.

In the first twelve months of my heart disease diagnosis, I continued with my executive role, meaning constant travel. This posed major barriers to maintaining my personal recovery.

Between hotel food, irregular schedules, and frequent flights, the only constant in my life was disruption. If I wanted to sustain my Mind, Body, and Soul, I had to build adaptability into my routine.

As a result, I developed a travel fitness strategy:

- Yoga in my hotel room before breakfast to keep my body engaged.
- Push-ups after my shower to maintain strength.
- Regulating my buffet selection to focus on fruit, vegetables, seafood, and nuts.
- Swimming or gym sessions twice a week, ensuring I only booked hotels with proper facilities.

Tracking my progress via my watch training statistics helped keep me accountable. These adjustments allowed me to maintain homeostasis despite constant change.

This taught me that barriers to alignment fitness aren't roadblocks, they are challenges

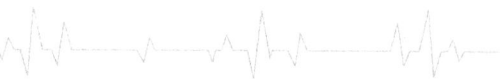

that require creative solutions. By adapting my approach, I ensured that Alignment Fitness remained part of my life, no matter the circumstances.

While I had built a strong foundation for Alignment Fitness, I soon realized that true progress required expert guidance and collaboration. At a certain point, self-directed training wasn't enough, as I'd discovered in other aspects of my journey, I needed professionals who could push me further while keeping me safe.

I worked with:

- A nutritionist to optimize dietary choices and support recovery.
- A fitness app tailored to my gym routine, refining my workouts based on my needs.
- A meditation coach to deepen my mindfulness practice and further integrate it into my daily routine.

Each expert helped me fine-tune my approach, ensuring that my physical, mental, and spiritual fitness remained in harmony. Collaboration wasn't about giving up control, it was about leveraging expertise to accelerate progress.

Alignment Fitness isn't about perfection, it's about progress.... The next chapter explores how to sustain progress over the long term by connecting with a network of fellow Titans.

Mind Fitness: Cultivating Clarity and Resilience

Fitness of the Mind focuses on emotional regulation, mental endurance, and clarity of thought. It requires intentional practices that promote mental flexibility and the capacity to handle life's uncertainties.

Key Practices for Mind Fitness:

- **Mindfulness and Meditation:** Center yourself in the present moment to reduce stress and increase focus.
- **Breathing Exercises:** Practice breathing techniques to reduce stress.
- **Cognitive Stimulation:** Engage in puzzles, problem-solving exercises, or creative activities to keep your mind sharp.
- **Emotional Processing:** Journaling or therapy can help you work through complex emotions tied to your diagnosis.

To enhance your progress, try pairing mental fitness practices with daily routines. For example, start the morning with a guided meditation or reflection, then take note of how it impacts your decision-making and emotional resilience throughout the day.

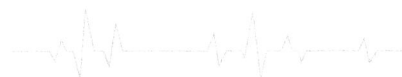

Body Fitness: Honoring Your Physical Needs

Physical fitness is not one-size-fits-all, especially for Titans managing chronic conditions. Alignment Body Fitness adapts to your current abilities while aiming to build strength, flexibility, and energy reserves.

Key Practices for Body Fitness:

- **Movement:** Low-impact exercises like yoga, swimming, or walking can be tailored to your needs.

- **Nutrition:** Partner with a dietitian to create a meal plan that supports your energy levels and overall health.

- **Rest and Recovery:** Incorporate adequate sleep and relaxation practices to allow your body to heal and rejuvenate.

Another way to personally improve is to listen to your body and honor its signals. Adjust routines based on fatigue levels, ensuring you balance exertion with rest.

Soul Fitness: Connecting with Purpose

The Soul represents your sense of meaning, connection, and joy. Soul Fitness is about nurturing this aspect of your alignment, whether through creative outlets, spiritual practices, or relationships.

Key Practices for Soul Fitness:

• **Spiritual Engagement:** Seek inspiration from your faith, belief system, or philosophy.

• **Community and Service:** Connect with others through shared values, volunteerism, or supportive relationships.

• **Creativity:** Explore activities that bring you joy, like painting, music, or journaling.

Wherever possible, schedule time for activities that nourish your Soul. Even small acts, like writing a gratitude list, can reconnect you with your values and purpose.

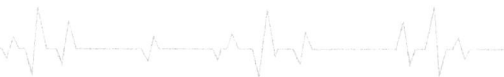

Dynamic Harmony in Alignment Fitness

True fitness arises when the Mind, Body, and Soul are balanced in a state of Dynamic Harmony. This means addressing the unique demands of your current situation while maintaining alignment across all three Elements.

Practical Applications:

• **Mind and Body Alignment:** Pair physical activity with mindfulness, such as a nature walk where you focus on sensory experiences.

• **Body and Soul Integration:** Choose movement practices that feel joyful, like dancing to your favorite music.

• **Mind and Soul Connection:** Reflect on how daily activities align with your values and bring a sense of fulfillment.

Barriers to Alignment Fitness and How to Overcome Them

Developing Alignment Fitness isn't without its challenges. Titans often encounter barriers like time constraints, fatigue, or fear of failure.

Strategies for Overcoming Barriers

• **Time Constraints:** Start small. Even five minutes of mindfulness or a brief stretch can make a difference.

• **Fatigue:** Prioritize restorative practices like hydration, gentle movement, and nutrition.

• **Fear of Failure:** Embrace the growth mindset by adding the word "yet" to your goals. For example, "I'm not there yet, but I'm making progress."

Alignment Fitness gives you a foundation. But even the strongest foundation needs direction and momentum to create lasting change. In the next chapter, we'll explore how small, consistent actions, built on presence, purpose, and alignment can help you sustain progress and move toward a future defined not by your diagnosis, but by your decisions.

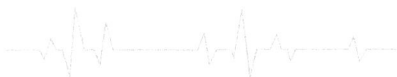

Key Insight

True fitness isn't just about how strong your body feels, it's about how aligned your mind, body, and soul are in facing each day with clarity, resilience, and purpose. Alignment Fitness is your lifelong practice of choosing alignment over perfection, one small action at a time.

Practical Reflections

As you begin to consider more than just physical fitness in your wellbeing routine it's time to consider the broader spectrum of Alignment Fitness.

- Which Element of your Alignment have you nurtured most this month?

- Inversely, which one have you been neglecting?

- What small routine can you build into your week to support that Element?

- Where can you combine strength and meaning bringing both joy and function to your wellbeing?

Fama's Sidebar

Your fitness journey is not about how fast or far you go, it's about how aligned you feel. Whether you're reaching out to a professional, stretching your body, or connecting with your purpose, every step forward counts. Remember, you don't have to do this alone, your team is here to help you thrive.

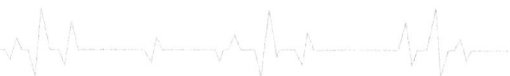

CHAPTER 16

Small Is Powerful

We often think transformation begins with a breakthrough, a dramatic moment that splits life into before and after. Yes, I'll agree that receiving a prostate disease, heart disease or cancer diagnosis is a big moment, and it is definitely a before and after scenario, but that's not how you rebuild, repair and live a life of reinvention.

Most of the Titans I've met, myself included, didn't find change in fireworks or speeches. We found it in *repetition*. In micro-decisions, in ordinary moments, and slight adjustments repeated with extraordinary intention.

Healing doesn't arrive in sweeping gestures.
It shows up as a glass of water.
A walk around the block.
A half smile.
A single, quiet "yes" to life.

The idea that change must be big, is one of the greatest myths holding people back from progress. In reality, the smallest steps are the most consistent builders of resilience, because they're the only ones we can actually take when the world feels heavy.

There are plenty of moments when I've felt I failed or slipped and they tend to happen in those moments of doubt just before I rock up to a progress evaluation of some kind. It happens in moments like the time I was heading to my annual TCM organ function test. My watch data was indicating a downward kick in my overall health. Not just in my overall health but my heart indicators and others were also trending down.

When I woke up that morning it felt like I was back to about eight or nine years old. For your reference, it was the 1970's and I was walking home from school one day when I found a magpie that had been hit by a car. It was still alive, but clearly needed help, visibly suffering from severe concussion or worse, brain damage. Mum and I spent months feeding and nursing Magpie back to health. In time it became quite tame and very friendly, often sitting on my hand like a pet while I fed it. Then, one morning I woke up and walked over to Magpies box only to find it had returned to a state of severe concussion with its head and eyes rolling around uncontrollably. Magpie died soon after.

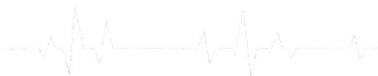

There are only a few dozen moments I remember from my childhood and that's one of them.

Come forward five decades to that morning in 2025 when I was sitting in the clinic waiting room, and that's how I felt about myself. Was I regressing? Was all this decoding stuff just rubbish created by a fanciful mind, thinking I could actually change the course of nature? Was I just like Magpie trying to beat the severe concussion of reality?

I received the TCM results. I had repaired myself to the level of being healthier than 83% of men my age. With the evaporation of doubt, I was back on the pathway of my empowered diagnosis, certainly not the outcome I expected but we always have to keep progressing forward, sorry Magpie.

I'm the first to admit I was the sort of person who focused on big changes, heck I was an entrepreneur, we have to think big or go home, but being diagnosed with a severe chronic condition changes your perspective entirely. All of a sudden you start focusing on small steps, small changes, small wins.

At the start of my heart crash of 2024, when the condition was at 40% health and falling fast, the first thing that crossed my mind was how do I stop myself falling off the cliff? I'd be dead in months if I didn't come up with something fast. But the more I thought of big changes, the more I understood there wasn't time. *Fast change meant small steps*. I first had to evaluate my decoding profile. Identify what the core issues were and work on each of them individually, starting with critical then working out to preferable.

Then, one small step at a time, first days, then by weeks and finally by months, I recovered but it wasn't from making huge gigantic leaps of change, it was by small incremental adjustments and I did it, my health recovered. I could write a book about those couple of months because the amount of change was significant but the only way to make significant change is by doing small things. In some instances those things were life changing, but it was all done one small step at a time and the end result of 'recovery' would not have happened without them.

When I think about those moments of intentional action and the dramatic recovery from my heart crash, there is one keystone habit that comes to mind and that's the habit of just showing up.

For decades now I've been talking the big talk, doing the big things but in reality, true success in life and in an empowered diagnosis is about showing up. During the prostate cancer treatment and now during the heart disease era I find the best results are by just doing small things as consistently as you can and as often as you can. What I mean, is being honest with yourself and not trying to smash big targets. This is not a game, this is your life so make it count.

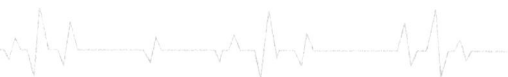

For instance, I don't meditate every morning but I do my best to do three or four every week and the peace of mind I maintain is enough. I'd love to do yoga every day to be the ultimate guru in flexibility, but in reality as long as I do two sessions a week and stretch the other days, then I know my inner core is being maintained and I'm less prone to injury as a result. When it comes to diet, it's the same imperfect regularity. Nearly every day starts with a fish and vege cook up with my standard medicinal smashed Avocado on Almond Road and fibre powders. Do I have it every day? No, but it's on the menu at least five mornings a week.

Just showing up every day, doing as many of my things, to the best of my ability at the time is a keystone habit that produces long term results over time, sending ripples of success well into my future.

Of course life has its ebbs and flows, and as Titans, we don't wake up every day full of zest and vitality. This morning for instance I woke up with a cracking headache. I really wasn't into doing anything. I looked into the kitchen and thought about breakfast, naaaaah, the thought of prepping food just didn't do it for me. I looked out the window and thought about a bike ride, naaaaah, it looked like rain. As my mind switched from activity to activity, nothing gelled. Stretches, no, meditation, heck no, with this headache? But then I started thinking about writing this chapter and asking myself how I was going to achieve that in this mental state.

Instead of dwelling on the lack of energy, the only clear answer, that kept resurfacing, was to take a couple of paracetamol and start somewhere. Coffee, I could brew coffee and that started the chain reaction. Before long the veggies were coming out of the fridge and onto the chopping board, then while my breakfast was cooking, it was time for my stretches and then even the vacuum cleaner came out and what started as a few pills to stave off lethargy ended up with twenty five push ups and chapter 16. Once again proving, it's the small steps that matter.

It's the gentleness of taking small steps, like swallowing a few paracetamol, not the force of making big changes, but leading with one step after the other that really makes the difference.

Just recently I did a strange thing. I gave myself a back injury doing Yoga. Yes I know, you can laugh at my expense, it's ok. My wife and I have been doing yoga for approximately fifteen years so you could say we are reasonably advanced, but there I was in class one evening, doing a Yin Yoga session and as I was coming out of a Turtle pose, my foot was asleep. Ok that's not unusual but after five minutes, then ten minutes, I began to wonder.

The visit to the Chiropractor the next day proved I had compressed the disc in my vertebrae where the spine joins the hip and the nervous system was impacted as a result. This would take months to repair and worst of all, all activity was out of bounds.

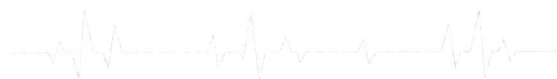

But what about exercise I thought? I had to stop everything physical, I couldn't drive and couldn't walk, and so had to embark on two months of recovery. As I write this chapter, I am still on the recovery path, but thanks to weekly visits to the chiropractor and more importantly, three half hour sessions per day of specific stretches I'm on the mend. Week by week I've improved and a few days ago I was able to return to balancing on the balls of my feet while brushing my teeth. Granted it was only a thirty second glimpse, but it was a small step and I knew by trying to pose a little longer every time I would soon be back to my two minute routine.

I'm not back on my bike, or able to go to the gym just yet, but I'm doing what I can to maintain my health and focus as best I can on constantly rehabilitating my foot, one step and one stretch at a time.

Small Alignments, Big Ripples

When we look through the lens of The Alignment Codex (as we did in the Introduction), micro-decisions function as alignment signals. Each one has a ripple effect:

- **Mind:** A decision to pause before reacting creates space for self-compassion.
- **Body:** A stretch, a breath, a moment of stillness calms the nervous system.
- **Soul:** A whispered prayer, a quiet "thank you," a step toward meaning.

These actions don't require fanfare. But they realign your decoding with precision and the ripple isn't theoretical, it's biological.

> *Neuroscience calls this habit stacking. Systems biology calls it feedback loops. We call it Dynamic Harmony.*

Because alignment isn't found in extreme effort, it's found in repeatable choices that honor who you are and what you need right now.

What the Codex Records

The Alignment Codex doesn't just record major breakthroughs. It's carved by the small. The subtle. The sacred.

It's carved by the moment you choose presence over panic or the choice to speak gently to your own fatigue and the decision to breathe before deciding.

These are not "lesser" steps. These are your foundation for change. Every small action, when done with intention, becomes an action in your *Alignment Codex*, proof that you showed up, recalibrated, and kept walking.

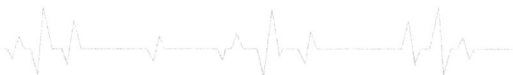

The Keystone Principle

In the field of behavior design, experts speak of 'keystone habits' or small actions that unlock broader transformation. These are the anchor points that, once installed, naturally lead to other changes.

For example:

- Drinking water in the morning often leads to better food decisions later.
- A 3-minute breath practice at lunch may reduce emotional reactivity in the afternoon.
- Writing one sentence in your journal can rewire your evening routine toward calm.

The goal is not *perfection*. It's *progress*. And keystone habits are how we get there, one act at a time.

Repair Is Also Power

There's a part of the journey we don't talk about enough: repair.

Not the heroic build. Not the shiny breakthrough. But the quiet moment after a misstep, where you choose to re-enter the path, even after slipping.

The truth is, alignment isn't lost in the fall. It's lost when we decide not to return.

And so much of your power as a Titan lies not in doing things perfectly, but in being willing to come back, to repair trust with your body, your mind, your habits. Not all at once. Not with guilt. But with small, sincere steps.

- One honest reflection.
- One choice to pause instead of punish.
- One moment where you say, "I'm still in this."

Recovery is a rhythm, resilience is a relationship and repair is a practice.

Your Codex doesn't expect perfection. It records participation.

When Small Is Sacred

There will be days when all you can do is breathe. When simply getting out of bed is a victory. Those moments are sacred, when your decoding feels fragmented and your energy feels gone.

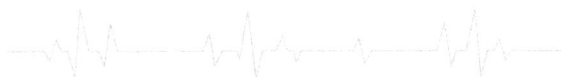

These are not failures, they are the most important days to choose small. Because it's in those moments, when we feel furthest from health, that alignment is most precious.

Small actions remind us that we are still participating. Still creating. Still walking.

And as long as you're still moving forward, you are not stuck.

Small Is a Strategy

In the end, small is not the consolation prize. It is the strategy.

It is how we build momentum. How we engage the present. How we decode a diagnosis is by progressing through one tiny act at a time.

Let go of the need for a heroic sprint, and choose a small, powerful step, today, now, right here on the Knife Edge of Time.

In the next chapter, we'll explore how to anchor those small, powerful choices in presence. Mindfulness isn't an escape, it's a return. A moment-to-moment invitation to notice, breathe, and recalibrate. You'll learn how to build mindfulness into your day, not as something you must schedule, but something you live.

Key Insight

The most profound change comes not from grand gestures, but from small, repeated acts of alignment. Repair, rebuild, and return, one step at a time.

Practical Reflections

- What's one small, repeatable choice that brings you back into alignment?

- What keystone habit could you introduce that might create positive ripples?

- Where in your journey have you slipped, and how did you (or could you) repair?

- What would "participation" look like for you today, even in its smallest form?

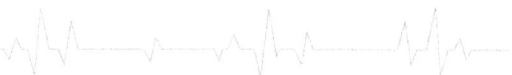

Fama's Sidebar: *The Return Is the Victory*

Don't wait for a grand comeback. The quiet act of returning, even after a misstep, is a triumph. Small choices realign you. A breath, a kind thought, a tiny action. This isn't about starting over. It's about continuing. Begin again. Right now.

CHAPTER 17

Establishing Mindfulness Practices

In a world that demands constant urgency, presence becomes a radical act. For Titans facing a chronic diagnosis like cancer or prostate disease, mindfulness isn't just a wellness trend or stress hack, it's survival. It is how we stay present, how we self-regulate, and how we align the Mind, Body, and Soul when everything feels like it's slipping out of sync.

During my journey with heart disease, I sought out multiple approaches to managing my stress and health. I had tried traditional meditation before, but nothing truly landed until I visited the Kanha Shanti Vanam ashram in India. It was there that I encountered a deeply embodied form of mindfulness, one that centred not just the mind, but the heart.

Heartfulness is an approach to meditation that focuses on inner stillness and clarity. During my time at the ashram, I practiced daily meditation, tuning into the subtle energy of my heart. The experience was transformative. For the first time, I felt a profound connection between my Mind, Body, and Soul in a way that words couldn't capture.

Upon returning home, I made meditation a part of my daily routine. It provided a sense of calm, clarity, and alignment that helped me navigate my health challenges with greater resilience. This practice reinforced a key decoding principle: mindfulness isn't just about managing stress, it's about cultivating a deep, ongoing relationship with yourself.

I'll admit, there were moments when the weight of my diagnosis felt unbearable. The uncertainty, the constant medical appointments, the lifestyle adjustments, it all compounded into a sense of overwhelming anxiety. However, one simple practice consistently brought me back to center: mindful breathing.

Each morning, before starting my day, I dedicated a few minutes to deep breathing. I would inhale for four counts, hold for four counts, and exhale for six. This rhythmic pattern slowed my heart rate, calmed my nervous system, and helped me approach the day with greater ease.

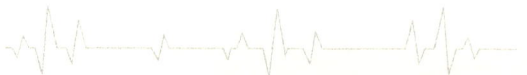

One day, while waiting for an important medical test, I felt my anxiety rising. My hands grew clammy, my heart raced, and my mind jumped to the worst-case scenario. Instead of spiraling, I closed my eyes and returned to my breath. Within moments, I felt my body relax, my mind clear, and my emotions stabilize. Mindful breathing became my go-to tool, helping me manage stress in real-time and reinforcing my ability to remain present and in control.

This chapter introduces mindfulness as a dynamic and accessible practice that integrates seamlessly with your decoding journey. Through reflective exercises, practical tools, and real-life examples, you will discover how mindfulness can become an anchor in your journey toward balance and empowerment.

Mindfulness

The Power of Presence

Mindfulness is the practice of bringing your attention to the present moment without judgment. Imagine standing in the eye of a storm, the chaos swirls around you, but within the center, there is stillness. Mindfulness allows you to find calm amidst life's turbulence, anchoring you in the now.

Being mindful and attaining presence in the moment has many benefits such as:
• Reducing mental clutter and stress.
• Enhances emotional regulation and clarity.
• Strengthens connection to the Body and Soul.

Building Awareness Through Mindfulness

Mindfulness has many connections to decoding such as:
• **Mind:** Cultivates mental clarity and reduces overthinking.
• **Body:** Increases awareness of physical sensations and needs.
• **Soul:** Deepens connection to purpose and joy.

Something to be aware of when practicing mindfulness are things like:
• Distractions, habitual thought patterns, and external pressures.
• Addressing the common challenges Titans face as a result of their condition when practicing mindfulness. (Try using a search engine to source these for your diagnosis)

Types of Mindfulness Practices

- **Breath Awareness:**
  - A foundational practice to anchor attention and regulate the nervous system.

- **Body Scanning:**
  - A practice to tune into physical sensations and identify areas of tension.

- **Mindful Movement:**
  - Incorporating mindfulness into walking, stretching, or other gentle activities.

- **Gratitude Practices:**
  - Using mindfulness to cultivate an attitude of gratitude and appreciation.

- **Meditative Visualization:**
  - Creating a mental sanctuary for calm and focus.

Practical Application

Over time, I developed a handful of go-to practices that brought me back to center. Here are three that became anchors for me...

Exercise 1: Breathing for Clarity

- Sit in a comfortable position and close your eyes.
- Take a slow, deep breath in through your nose, counting to four.
- Hold your breath for a count of four.
- Exhale slowly through your mouth, counting to six.
- Repeat for five cycles, focusing solely on your breath.

Exercise 2: Body Scan for Awareness

- Lie down or sit comfortably in a quiet space.
- Starting at your toes, bring your attention to each part of your body, moving upward.
- Notice any sensations, tension, or discomfort without judgment.
- Conclude the scan by focusing on your breath for two minutes.

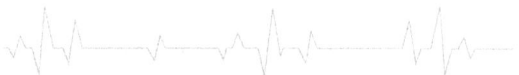

Exercise 3: Mindful Walking

- Choose a quiet space for a short walk.
- Focus on the sensation of your feet touching the ground with each step.
- Observe your surroundings, the sounds, sights, and smells without judgment.
- Reflect on how this practice centers your thoughts and calms your body.

Movement had always been part of my recovery process, but in the past, I had treated exercise as a task rather than an experience. That changed when I reframed my daily walks as mindfulness rituals.

Instead of walking with distractions, listening to podcasts, scrolling through my phone, or planning my next task, I chose to walk with presence. I paid attention to the sensation of my feet hitting the ground, the rhythm of my breath, the sounds of nature around me. Each step became a meditation, an opportunity to tune into my surroundings and reconnect with myself.

This simple shift transformed my daily routine. It made movement feel purposeful, nourishing, and restorative. More importantly, it reinforced a central lesson: mindfulness isn't something separate from life, it is something to be woven into the fabric of everything we do.

In those walks we don't just exercise, we refresh and align.

Once we begin to cultivate presence, we start to hear things more clearly, our longings, our values, our internal compass. In the next chapter, we explore the role of spirituality in healing and how connecting with something larger than yourself can bring deep resilience to your decoding journey.

Key Insight

Mindfulness isn't a retreat from life, it's a return to it. Presence aligns your decoding and restores clarity, one breath at a time.

Practical Reflection Prompts

- What distractions most often pull you away from the present moment?
- When you feel scattered, what's one small practice that helps you return?
- How does mindful awareness influence your connection to your body's needs?
- When was the last time you paused long enough to hear the whisper of your Soul?
  a. What did it say?
- How can you turn an everyday activity (e.g. walking, eating, showering) into a mindfulness ritual?

Fama's Sidebar
Mindfulness in Action

Mindfulness isn't about clearing your mind, it's about coming home to it. Each time you choose presence over distraction, you realign your dynamic harmony.

Start small: one breath, one step, one moment of awareness. You don't need stillness to begin, you need only to begin.

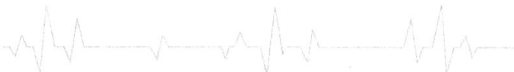

CHAPTER 18

Exploring Spirituality

Life often feels like a rushing river, unpredictable and relentless. But within this flow lies stillness, a quiet strength that allows us to move with, rather than against, the current.

The Tao Te Ching describes this balance as harmony with the natural flow of existence, while Heartfulness Yoga offers tools to quiet the mind and open the heart. For Titans navigating chronic conditions, this harmony of both of these ancient philosophies nurture resilience, purpose, and alignment.

Spirituality doesn't need to fit into a specific tradition or belief. In fact, for Titan's, we are referring to your spirit or essence of life rather than any ritual or tradition you follow as a religion. Exploring spirituality is about discovering what brings meaning to your life.

So where does one start?

The Tao's wisdom and Heartfulness practices can be a great start to guide one toward connection, balance, and purpose.

Life with a chronic condition like cancer often feels isolating, pulling you away from a sense of self and purpose. Yet spirituality offers a bridge back to wholeness, inviting you to reconnect with your inner strength and the greater flow of life.

The Tao's Perspective: The Tao teaches that life's essence lies in accepting and flowing with what is, rather than resisting. It invites us to embrace imperfection and trust the process.

Key Wisdom: "The wise do not force; they flow with the universe.".

Heartfulness Insight: Heartfulness meditation emphasizes connecting to the heart as a source of calm and clarity, allowing you to navigate life's uncertainties with grace.

At the onset of my heart disease diagnosis, I struggled with the idea of slowing down. I had spent a lifetime thriving on productivity, equating busyness with success. The thought of surrendering control to an illness felt impossible, and the same applied during the prostate disease diagnosis. Resistance became my default response, resistance to change, to limitation, to the idea that I might not have full command over my future.

But resistance itself became a source of stress. It wasn't until I started practicing heartfulness meditation that I realized how much energy I was expending fighting what I couldn't change. Through meditation, I began to shift my perspective. Instead of viewing adaptation as defeat, I reframed it as an opportunity for growth. Releasing resistance didn't mean giving up, it meant making space for healing, for acceptance, for a new way forward.

A friend later told me, "Health is your new occupation." That simple statement changed a lot for me. Instead of treating my recovery as a secondary task, I began to view it as my primary focus. My mindset shifted from managing illness to actively occupying health. This reframing gave me a renewed sense of purpose, aligning perfectly with the decoding philosophy. I wasn't just reacting to the condition, I was actively shaping my wellbeing, making intentional choices that honored my Mind, Body, and Soul.

Before my heart disease diagnosis, I had a rigid idea of what success looked like. I measured my worth by achievements, by pushing harder, by always being in motion. But illness forced me to slow down, and in doing so, I was confronted with the discomfort of stillness.

Instead of pushing I went in the other direction, slowing down and starting each day with a half-hour Heartfulness meditation as a way to connect my Mind, Body, and Soul. Instead of approaching my practice with the expectation of achieving a specific outcome, I allowed myself to simply be present. As I moved through breath control, concentration, and meditation, I found an unexpected ease. For the first time I wasn't battling my limitations, I was aligning with them, flowing through each moment rather than resisting it.

This lesson extended beyond that single walk. I began applying the same principle to my daily life, allowing room for flow instead of forcing rigid expectations. My journey didn't have to follow a predetermined map; I could navigate with flexibility, adjusting as needed. In surrendering to the present moment, I found ease where I once found struggle.

When I made the decision to have a penile implant after prostate cancer surgery, I struggled with what it meant for my masculinity and identity. It wasn't just a medical procedure; it was a fundamental shift in how I viewed myself. I needed a way to process this change, so I began journaling what I called my 'Life Force Entries.'

At first, these entries were scattered thoughts, frustrations, fears, and doubts. But over time, they evolved into something deeper: a record of resilience, discovery, and self-acceptance. Each entry became a reflection on not just my physical state but my emotional and spiritual well-being. Writing gave me a way to reclaim my sense of self beyond the diagnosis.

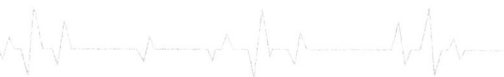

Through this practice, I realized that purpose wasn't about what I had lost but about what I could still create. My journal became a testament to my ability to adapt and evolve, reminding me that purpose exists not in perfection but in the small, deliberate steps we take toward self-acceptance and growth.

One challenge I faced in my spiritual journey was reconciling seemingly opposing truths. I was deeply grateful for the life I still had, yet I also mourned the parts of me that illness had changed. I felt strong in my ability to navigate my diagnosis, yet vulnerable in the face of uncertainty. It was an internal struggle that seemed impossible to resolve.

Through meditation and reflection, I came to understand that balance doesn't mean eliminating struggle, it means learning to hold both realities at once. I could grieve and still be grateful. I could feel uncertain and still move forward with confidence. This realization became a cornerstone of my spiritual practice, teaching me that true resilience isn't about choosing one state over another, but embracing the duality of life.

As I continued this practice, I found a sense of peace not in answers, but in acceptance. Holding opposites in balance allowed me to move forward without needing to fix or change everything, and that shift in perspective became one of the most powerful tools in my healing journey.

One profound shift in my journey came when I recognized that true healing required more than just addressing my physical condition, it demanded a deeper connection with myself and those around me. It wasn't until I embraced heartfulness meditation and truly listened to my inner voice that I understood what I had been missing.

During one particular meditation session, I felt an overwhelming sense of presence, as if all the barriers I had built between myself and the world dissolved. For the first time, I wasn't just existing with my diagnosis, I was integrating it into my life, making peace with the uncertainty. This newfound connection expanded beyond myself. It transformed my relationships, allowing me to be more open, more vulnerable, and more present with those I loved.

Through this experience, I learned that spirituality isn't just about finding answers; it's about embracing the unknown with trust and acceptance. The deepest connection isn't to an outcome but to the journey itself, and in that realization, I found a profound sense of peace.

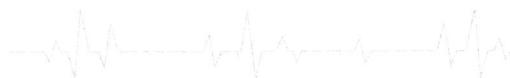

The Path to Purpose

Purpose is not a grand destination, it's found in the small, meaningful moments that remind us of our connection to the world. Here's how the Tao and Heartfulness can illuminate this path:

Surrender and Acceptance

- The Tao: The Tao emphasizes "Wu Wei" (effortless action), which teaches that surrendering to life's flow allows for harmony.
- Heartfulness: Heartfulness cleaning techniques clear the mind and heart of burdens, making space for calm acceptance.

Finding Meaning in Stillness

- The Tao: "Stillness reveals the true path.". In quiet moments, the heart reveals clarity and purpose.
- Heartfulness: Silent meditation centers you in the present, opening a space for reflection and deeper connection.

Living with Harmony and Duality

- The Tao: Life's dualities (light/dark, joy/sorrow) are essential for balance. True dynamic harmony comes from accepting both and allowing the balance to come and go between them.
- Heartfulness: The heart has the capacity to hold vulnerability and strength simultaneously, fostering resilience.

Practical Application

Merging Philosophy with Practice

A Tao-Inspired Heartfulness Meditation

- Sit comfortably and imagine a river representing life's flow.
- Let your breath mirror the river steady and smooth.
- Bring your awareness to your heart. Visualize it as a still, reflective pool within the river and from that pool emanates your divine light or being.

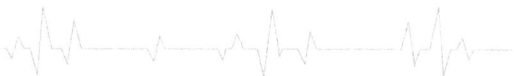

Heartfulness Cleaning for Release

- At the end of your day, recall any burdens or tensions.
- Visualize them dissolving in light and being drawing through your body and out through your back as wafts of smoke.
- If a thought enters your mind, don't hold it, don't interrogate it, just let it go.
- Cleansing your thoughts leaves your heart lighter and more open to explore your source.

Journaling Notes

- Each evening, write down three small moments of gratitude. Reflect on how they nurture your connection to purpose.

Key Insight

- The Tao Te Ching and Heartfulness Yoga share a focus on surrender, balance, and inner wisdom.

- Spirituality reconnects Titans with their Soul, providing resilience and clarity.

- Consistent practices like meditation, journaling, and cleaning foster alignment and purpose.

With a stronger connection to your Soul, the next step is aligning your lifestyle choices with The Alignment Pathway. In the following chapter, we'll explore how daily decisions and habits can reinforce alignment and support your growth.

Fama's Sidebar
Aligning with the Flow

Spirituality is your compass, guiding you to align with life's flow. The Tao reminds us to let go and trust the journey, while Heartfulness teaches us to listen deeply to the wisdom within. Today, pause and ask yourself: What does my heart need right now? Trust its guidance—it always leads you home.

CHAPTER 19

Overcoming Limiting Beliefs

Overcoming limiting beliefs may be the kickstart you need to begin your Alignment Pathway.

For me, self-doubt related to the incurable heart disease was a major limiting factor that held me back. Upon reflection, I'm amazed at how much valuable restorative time I wasted by letting self-doubt consume me before I actually shook it off. It took me three months from diagnosis to my first action.

I had fallen into a spiral of internalized fear. The thought of an "incurable" condition became a mental weight, making every step forward feel futile. My inner critic fueled the narrative that there was no point in trying, that heart disease had already determined my future. I convinced myself that no matter what I did, the outcome wouldn't change.

It wasn't until my wife noticed a shift in my demeanor that she suggested I talk to a psychologist. That single step changed everything. After multiple sessions, I was diagnosed with depression, something I later learned is a common early-stage symptom of a life-altering diagnosis like heart disease.

I was allowing the word incurable to dictate my mindset, feeding the very self-doubt that was stopping me from acting. My psychologist helped me reframe my perspective, breaking down the overwhelming idea of "curing" the condition into manageable, progressive steps. Instead of focusing on what I couldn't control, I shifted my energy toward what I could starting with small, consistent changes.

Once I reframed my thinking, my pathway opened up. I began implementing incremental goals, first with diet, then movement, then structured daily habits. With every small win, my self-doubt weakened. Within months, I had regained control of my outlook, replacing uncertainty with determination.

The lesson? The greatest barrier to progress wasn't the condition, it was my belief about the condition. And once I changed that, I changed everything.

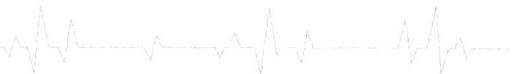

Overcoming these beliefs creates dynamic harmony across your Trinity, empowering you to take aligned actions to support growth and resilience.

In my case, the fear of failure showed up in the lead-up to my prostate cancer surgery.

The thought of living with erectile dysfunction terrified me. I recall sitting in the pre-operative room, waiting for my turn, looking at the door and contemplating an escape. I knew I couldn't leave, but the fear was almost unbearable.

Even before arriving at the hospital, waves of anxiety had washed over me. I was grappling with thoughts of masculinity, identity, and the permanence of what was about to happen. My inner dialogue was relentless: Would I still be the same? Would my marriage suffer? Was I making the wrong choice?

I had spent countless hours researching alternative treatments, grasping at anything that might allow me to avoid surgery. But deep down, I knew I had exhausted all options, this was the best course of action for my long-term survival. The reality was, my fear of failure wasn't about the surgery itself, it was about what life would look like after it.

Reframing my perspective became the key to overcoming that fear. Yes, my sex life was going to change, but that didn't mean it was over. In fact, it became an opportunity for my wife and me to explore new methods of intimacy. Through medical consultations, I learned about options like penile implants and targeted therapies, reassuring me that I wasn't out of options.

By shifting from a fear of loss to an openness to adaptation, I moved forward with confidence. I went into surgery knowing that while some things would be different, my ability to create joy, connection, and intimacy remained within my control.

There was a moment during my heart disease journey when I almost lost my motivation to keep fighting.

I was sitting in my Traditional Chinese Medicine (TCM) clinic, waiting for my first annual review since my heart disease diagnosis. I felt utterly defeated. My heart score had plummeted by 20% in four weeks, erasing months of progress. It was a crushing blow.

I remember thinking: What's the point? I'm fighting a losing battle.

But then, as I reviewed my overall health report with my TCM doctor, something astonishing happened. My overall wellness score, measured by meridian energy assessment, was at an all-time high. Not just a slight improvement, but an unprecedented 8% increase.

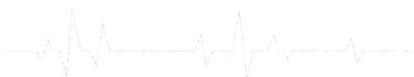

In that moment, I realized something powerful: progress isn't always linear, and it's not always visible. While my heart health had fluctuated, my overall well-being had improved dramatically.

That shift in perspective reignited my sense of purpose. Instead of obsessing over isolated data points, I began focusing on sustaining health as an occupation, rather than an endless battle. This wasn't just about managing heart disease, it was about creating a thriving, fulfilling life.

I had been so fixated on numbers that I had forgotten the bigger picture: I was healthier than I had ever been in my adult life, and I needed to own that. That realization changed the trajectory of my journey.

Breaking Free from Mental Chains

Limiting beliefs are the invisible barriers that keep Titans from embracing their full potential. These beliefs often stem from past experiences, societal expectations, or self-doubt. They whisper fears like "I can't do this," or "I'm not enough." But the truth is, these beliefs are not facts, they're stories. And just as they were created, they can be rewritten.

Let's identify the limiting beliefs holding you back, challenge them with evidence, and replace them with empowering truths. By transforming your mindset, you'll unlock new possibilities and strengthen your alignment with decoding, Mind, Body, and Soul. Together, we'll turn those whispers of doubt into declarations of strength and resilience.

The Guide: The Role of Limiting Beliefs in Decoding Your Diagnosis

Every limiting belief disrupts your decoding in unique ways:

- **Mind:** Creates mental loops of self-doubt or defeat, clouding decision-making and fostering fear.
  - **Example:** "I can't manage this diagnosis" overwhelms the Mind and blocks problem-solving.

- **Body:** Discourages aligned actions, such as seeking treatment or prioritizing self-care.
  - **Example:** "I don't have the energy for this" leads to inaction, depleting physical vitality.

- **Soul:** Disconnects you from purpose and joy, fostering feelings of hopelessness or emptiness.
  - **Example:** "I don't deserve to feel better" isolates the Soul from fulfillment.

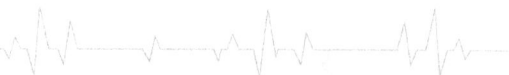

The Problem: Identifying the Limiting Beliefs Holding You Back

Limiting beliefs often masquerade as truths, making them difficult to recognize. They may sound like:

- "I'm not strong enough to overcome this challenge."
- "If I ask for help, it means I'm weak."
- "I've failed before, so I'll fail again."

These beliefs act as roadblocks, keeping you from fully engaging with The Alignment Pathway. But identifying them is the first step to rewriting the narrative.

Key Insights

- Limiting beliefs disrupt alignment, creating imbalance across the Mind, Body, and Soul.

- By identifying and reframing these beliefs, you can restore harmony and unlock new possibilities.

- Empowering beliefs inspire aligned actions, fostering resilience and growth.

The truth is, your condition does not define you. Your beliefs do. And once you shift them, you shift everything.

As you let go of limiting beliefs, you make space to celebrate your progress and embrace your wins.

In the next chapter, we'll explore the importance of honoring your journey and finding joy in every milestone, no matter how small.

Practical Reflections

Challenging Limiting Beliefs

1. Identify the Belief: Write down one belief that feels restrictive (e.g., "I'll never be able to change.").
2. Challenge It: Reflect on evidence that proves this belief wrong. Think of past successes or strengths you've demonstrated.
3. Reframe It: Rewrite the belief in a way that empowers you (e.g., "Change is possible, and I am capable of taking small, meaningful steps forward.").
4. Take Action: Choose one action today that aligns with this new belief.

Rewriting Your Narrative

- Reflect on a time when a limiting belief held you back. How did it impact your actions or choices?

- Imagine how reframing that belief might have changed the outcome. What empowering belief can you adopt moving forward?

Fama's Sidebar: Transforming Limiting Beliefs

Every belief you hold is like a stepping stone or a roadblock on your journey. Which beliefs are helping you move forward, and which ones are keeping you stuck? Today, I invite you to challenge one limiting belief. Reframe it into a truth that supports your growth. Remember, every small shift in perspective opens the door to big transformations.

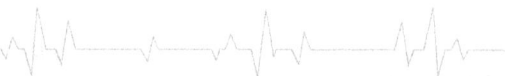

CHAPTER 20

Health Is Your Occupation

Reframing post-diagnosis life as a craft or vocation.

My wife and I had just returned to Brisbane after three weeks of work-related travel that began with an abrupt and unforeseen end to her senior role in the organisation. That was followed by me co-hosting a conference in the Cook Islands, then returning to Sydney to serve as one of the CEOs at our corporate annual conference.

I won't unpack every detail of those three weeks, but by the time we returned to Brisbane, I was mentally, physically, and spiritually exhausted.

We weren't even going home, we were house-sitting my parents' apartment overlooking Brisbane city and the Story Bridge. It should have been relaxing, but I couldn't shake the sense that something had to change.

I was juggling two worlds, and the stress was too much. My wife noticed my pale complexion and said I didn't 'look myself'. I called the independent corporate therapy line to talk through my concerns. After days of counselling, the truth was clear: I had to make a dramatic change or my heart condition would do it for me, possibly in the worst way.

This was the moment I spoke about in earlier chapters during the heart disease causing a dramatic decline. But this chapter isn't about the crash. It's about what happened next.

In the months of rehabilitation, it became clear that health was something I had been neglecting for decades. That had to stop if I was to survive beyond Christmas. Those first few weeks felt like sliding down an icy cliff toward death, an image I never forgot. I had to move away from that cliff, fast.

You might think; easy, just exercise more. But decoding a chronic diagnosis like cancer or heart disease means achieving alignment across mind, body, and soul. That's not something you dabble in. It takes vocational-level commitment.

A few months later, my wife and I went on a day sail aboard the ship where I once served as Sailing Master. My old friend Neil, was the master that day. We hadn't seen each other in years, so we spent the trip reminiscing. I gave him the short version of my health journey.

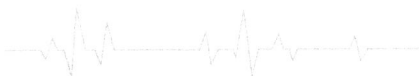

He listened, then said, "Health is your new occupation."

It landed with the weight of truth. My health wasn't a job I could clock in and out of, it was a vocation I had to commit to with discipline, curiosity, and skill. If I took it seriously, I could not only survive beyond my original prognosis but thrive for decades.

It was easy to take Neil's off-hand comment and treat it as a revelation, but what would it mean in practice?

- **Mind:** I had to learn about more my conditions, understand how they overlapped, and identify the risks that applied to all of them. At the top of the list was stress management which meant building awareness of triggers and reframing my identity. It took nearly a year of reflection, discussion, and "aha" moments to learn how to manage stress without withdrawing from life. My strongest suggestion: get professional help. A good therapist can be a master craftsman for the mental side of alignment.

- **Body:** Medication management, nutrition, exercise, rest cycles, and physical therapy were all essential, but rest was my biggest challenge. My days were packed: exercise, eating well, work, writing this book, and family time which meant rest got squeezed out, and fatigue took over.

- **Soul:** Purpose, connection, emotional resilience, and meaning beyond the diagnosis. This was the hardest element to understand, and to sustain. When you're in the thick of treatment, the diagnosis consumes everything. Once the medical focus stabalises, you have to redefine who you are, what matters, and where you're going.

The Craft of Stabilisation

Treating your health as your occupation means adopting the mindset of a skilled tradesperson or artisan. You're building mastery over time.

Daily "tasks" of this craft include:

- **Routines as non-negotiables:** Morning movement, medication, mindful eating, and rest are scheduled like important meetings.
- **Tracking progress without obsession:** Regular check-ins help you adapt without getting lost in numbers. Unfortunately I love data analysis so often get lost in analysis paralysis.
- **Seeking mentorship:** Specialists, therapists, support groups and casual mentors, these are your "professional network."
- **Continuing education:** Learn your body's signals and how they change with stress, diet, and environment.

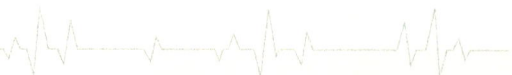

- **Practising Dynamic Harmony:** Adjusting your workload, activity, and expectations based on your daily capacity.

The Transition Point

This full-time health occupation doesn't have to last forever. For most people, the goal is to graduate, to move from constant vigilance into integrated maintenance.

With stability, the practices you learned become part of your life without dominating it. You can shift attention back to your career, hobbies, and adventures without letting health slide into the background.

Common Pitfalls

- **Treating health like a side hustle:** Trying to squeeze it into leftover time.

- **Overloading yourself:** Taking on every wellness strategy at once, then burning out.

- **Dropping the routine too soon:** Stopping healthy habits the moment you feel better.

Key Insight

In the early stages after diagnosis, your health is your full-time job. The more intentionally you commit to it, the sooner you can integrate it back into a balanced life.

Practical Reflections

- What would it look like to give your health the same structure and priority as your work?
- Which daily practices are truly non-negotiable for you right now?
- Where can you simplify to free up the energy for recovery?

Fama's Side Bar

Think of this as an apprenticeship with your own self. The skills you learn now will serve you for life long after the intensity of this season has passed.

CHAPTER 21

Do You Have a Chronic Travel Condition?

I do. Mine's an itch that demands scratching every six months. If I can't travel, I may as well be dead. As far as I'm concerned, Prostate Disease, Cancer or heart Disease are not going to stop me.

As Paul Cobbin 1.0, travel was never ordinary: walking through live minefields in the Atacama Desert, diving the Pandora wreck in search of Bounty mutineers, even being a mutineer myself. After meeting my wife, the pace didn't slow, unless you call backpacking across Vietnam with our teenage daughters or getting tear gassed in a Middle East refugee camp "slowing down."

This chapter isn't long enough for all those stories, maybe someday I publish them as a travelogue for Titans. Here in this chapter, I'll compare two journeys; one before diagnosis and one after, and the adjustments you might consider for your own travels.

Before Diagnosis: The Outer Landscape

Before my heart diagnosis, my wife and I hiked two weeks through Japan's Kii Mountains on the UNESCO-listed Kumano Kodo pilgrimage. Picture the samurai era: tight ravines, cedar forests, deep gorges, crystal rivers, and Shiro castles rising through mist. Rivers of cloud spilled over the ridges, jungle fog filled the valleys.

Stone steps, hundreds to over a thousand in a day linked remote villages. On the ascent to Hosshinmon-oji, we climbed 1,200 steps before lunch. We'd also done the Portuguese and Spanish Caminos. In hindsight, the Kumano Kodo was the riskiest; one way in, one way out, yet I hiked on, blissfully unaware that I was the last person who should have been doing it.

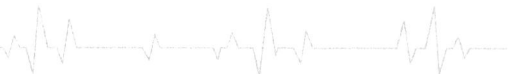

After Diagnosis: The Inner Landscape

Six months after my initial heart disease diagnosis, we travelled to India, to Kanha Shanti Vanam: 1,400 acres of gardens, meditation halls, and quiet walking paths.

We stayed in the Ayurvedic wellness centre, following a daily rhythm of sunrise meditation with thousands in the grand hall, vegetarian breakfast, then up to the college for asana yoga. Afternoons meant walking under tree-lined paths to lectures on the eight limbs of yoga, far more than the single asana most studios teach.

Then came the magic; Ayurvedic treatments.

In the quiet treatment room, a brass vessel swayed almost imperceptibly above the massage table, pouring a warm, herbal-infused stream of oil across my forehead traversing the "third eye." The heat sank into my scalp, thoughts dissolving into the rhythmic sound of oil on skin, the air rich with sesame and calming herbs.

Evenings ended with meditation in the gardens with the last light catching the golden statue of Babuji. The pace was restorative, the focus inward and a complete contrast to the Kumano's relentless forward motion.

Rethinking Travel with Chronic Conditions

At diagnosis, I wondered if I'd travel again. Would a four-hour hop to Fiji be possible, let alone halfway across the world? The answer was yes if I adapted.

Some hobbies were out for sure, like sailing 120-foot ships or scuba diving, but boundaries could shift. Coastal sailing with my wife? Yes. Ocean crossings? No. Highlands of Papua New Guinea or the Kokoda Track, where medical help is days away? Also no.

Instead, we seek adventures with manageable risk like spiritual retreats, cultural immersions and journeys with contingency plans. For a Himalayan meditation retreat, we'll prepare with peak fitness, pace our days, and slot in rest days between excursions.

Insurance

It is important you consult with your insurance provider (either anonymously or as the premium holder) to ascertain whether you have sufficient cover for the travelling in question. The nature of the policy describes it's limitations and I am not about to offer legal advice on insurance terminology.

However I will say it is important for your safety, not just the coverage.

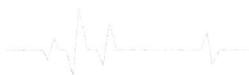

Consider the trip and a worst case scenario and the possibility of an event occurring. Once you have done that, ask yourself if the insurance policy will cover the event. If your response is "unsure" or "no", I suggest you consider either increasing the policy to cover the event, or seek an alternative insurer.

Pacing & Planning

We avoid back-to-back day trips, choosing a few highlights and using the rest for writing, exercise, or reflection. For Australians, overseas means long flights, so we break them with stopovers in Asia or the Middle East heading west, Hawaii or Fiji heading east. This slows the pace, reduces fatigue, and lowers risk.

Keep your daily routines intact. For me: a vegetarian breakfast with omega-3-rich fish on the side, and avoiding foods I wouldn't eat at home. Before diagnosis, I gained a kilo a week travelling; now, I stay stable.

Sleep hygiene is crucial so adjust your body clock before travel if possible, or allow rest days on arrival. Jet lag hits hardest eastbound, so I plan quiet days at home upon return because if you are like me, you try to forge on and jump straight back into it the next day. I used to but now I don't. For me, travel fatigue can trigger heart palpitations so cramming too much into short trips increases medical risk.

Flying Responsibly

I don't drink alcohol, but if you do, avoid it while flying. Cabin air dehydrates you; alcohol accelerates it. Combine that with immobility, and your risk of deep vein thrombosis (DVT), already higher with chronic conditions, risk goes up. DVT leading to pulmonary embolism or cardiac arrest is the most common medical event on long-haul flights for people like us.

Arrive at your destination in the best condition so you can enjoy it.

On the Ground

Avoid unnecessary physical or mental stress, but keep moving through walking tours, cycling, local swims. I always pack goggles, cap, and swimmers or hire a bicycle. Exercising in another country, surrounded by locals, can be as memorable as any sightseeing.

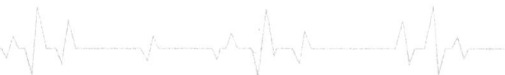

Medication Management

Preparation is key. I keep at least one week of spare medication in my wife's bag and vice versa, plus another week in my carry-on. For longer or remote trips, I pack extra. If COVID-style lockdowns taught us anything, it's that plans can change fast.

Carry a GP letter listing your prescriptions as it helps local doctors find the correct equivalent if needed. Brand names vary, but an ingredient list travels well.

Sleep

We've covered sleep in previous chapters in terms of alignment fitness and the same goes here with travel fitness. You sleep will be disrupted, there is no doubt about it. There are all sorts of forces impacting on your travel sleep such as, time zones differences, diet changes, new surroundings, changed bed comfort and different noises to assimilate.

You can't avoid these disruptors but you can reduce them by remembering your eye mask, taking ear plugs and if you have sleep apnea, taking a travel capable CPAP machine. With CPAP machines ensure the water you use in the humidifier is bottle water or you may find similar concerns as you would if you drink unfiltered water with stomach disorders.

Other methods I try to employ include limiting my bedside reading, meditating before sleep and relaxing music if ear plugs are not available.

Key Insight

Travelling with a chronic condition isn't about giving up the journeys you love, it's about reshaping them to fit the body you have now. Boundaries aren't the end of adventure; they're the framework that keeps the adventure sustainable.

Whether it's a meditative retreat or a mountain pilgrimage, the value of travel comes from engagement, presence, and connection, not the distance covered or the difficulty endured.

Practical Reflections

Know your limits and your boundaries
- Some trips are worth the extra planning; others aren't worth the risk. Decide early so you can focus on safe, rewarding options.

Pace your adventures
- Build in rest days, avoid back-to-back excursions, and allow time to adjust to new time zones.

Keep your routines intact
- Diet, exercise, medication, and sleep habits matter just as much on the road as at home.

Plan for contingencies
- Carry extra medication in separate bags, plus a doctor's letter with prescriptions listed by active ingredient.

Fly responsibly
- Hydrate, move often, and avoid alcohol to reduce DVT risk. Break long trips into segments where possible.

Look for joy in new forms
- If certain activities are no longer possible, seek experiences that offer the same sense of fulfilment in different ways.

Fama's Insight

A compass works the same whether you're crossing a mountain pass or walking a garden path. The key is knowing which direction serves you now. Your journey hasn't ended, it's simply taken a wiser route.

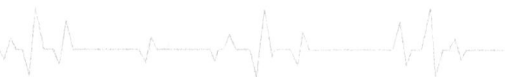

CHAPTER 22

Celebrating Progress and Wins

The road of life can feel long and winding, especially when navigating a chronic diagnosis. But even on the hardest days, there are moments of light we see as small victories that remind us of how far we've come. These moments, however fleeting, deserve celebration. They're not just milestones; they're fuel for the soul, proof of resilience, and reminders of the strength that lies within you.

In the early days of managing my heart disease diagnosis, I found myself overwhelmed by the enormity of the challenge ahead. It felt like I was climbing a mountain without ever catching sight of the peak. But instead of fixating on the summit, I started focusing on each step as small, incremental goals that reinforced my progress.

One of my biggest motivators became my health improvement score, an aggregate measurement from my smart devices that combined my heart rate, activity levels, and sleep quality. In October 2023, that score was at 60% and far from where I wanted it to be. By setting short, achievable targets, I gradually improved it to 74% by March 2024. The consistency of these small wins fueled my drive to push further.

The ripple effect of tracking progress became clear. Seeing even modest improvements motivated me to sustain healthy habits, reinforcing my commitment to The Alignment Pathway. By February 2025, my score peaked at 82% and eventually stabilized at 75% and remains so plus or minus a percent currently at 74% coming out of the Australian Winter, August 2025, a testimonial win to the power of persistence and consistency.

The lesson? Success isn't about giant leaps, it's about steady steps. By celebrating small wins, you create a positive feedback loop that fuels long-term progress.

There's something profound about achieving a long-term goal, one that requires years of discipline, setbacks, and unwavering commitment.

For me, one of the longest-standing milestones I have chased was raising my general health score to match that of a person *without* chronic disease.

In 2019, when I first took an organ health test, my result was 68%, a score below average for men my age. The test, which assessed my overall physiological function, made it painfully clear that I was on a downward trajectory.

Fast forward to January 2025 some six years later. After countless adjustments in nutrition, exercise, and stress management, I retook the same test. This time, the result was 83% which was a rating that placed me in the *excellent* category for men my age, regardless of chronic conditions.

That single number validated years of effort. It reinforced the idea that, despite my diagnosis, I had not only stopped the decline but reversed it.

The takeaway? Big wins come from thousands of small intentional choices. And when you reach a long-term milestone, take a moment to celebrate because it's proof of your resilience.

For me, celebrating became second nature and where possible I recorded my wins as Lifeforce Entries to reflect upon now as a 'lessons learnt' process and for future reflection to gauge progress. Some days, the win was monumental. Other days, it was as simple as, "I got out of bed." Both were equally worthy of celebration.

Progress isn't just measured in numbers; sometimes, the biggest victories are internal.

For years, my identity was tied to my job description and KPI's. Work was my purpose, my validation, and my drive. But when my heart disease diagnosis forced me to step down from my position, I found myself adrift.

The transition was brutal. I equated stepping away with failure, and for months, I wrestled with feelings of inadequacy. But over time, I realized that success wasn't about holding a title, it was about holding onto purpose.

I began celebrating non-traditional wins:
- Prioritizing my health without guilt.
- Rebuilding my life with intention.
- Finding fulfillment beyond my career.

> *"The greatest win of all? Learning that self-worth isn't tied to external validation, it's an inside job."*

For a long time, I measured my progress solely through outcomes in numbers, milestones, and external validation. I thought that success was something I would only feel after I reached a goal. But as I deepened my Alignment Pathway journey, I realized that joy doesn't come at the finish line, instead, it's found along the way.

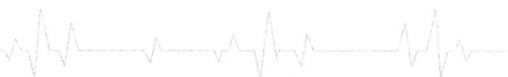

One of the biggest shifts in my perspective came when I started practicing gratitude daily. Instead of waiting for a major achievement to feel fulfilled, I began celebrating the simple things:

- The feeling of strength after a morning walk.
- The satisfaction of a nutritious, well-balanced meal.
- The quiet contentment of an uninterrupted, restful night's sleep.

By shifting my focus from where I wanted to be to where I was, I found more peace, more resilience, and, surprisingly, even better long-term results. When I stopped chasing joy and started cultivating joy daily, everything changed.

You'll notice a lot of positive changes, in my own path, throughout the book and there are two suggestions in this one reflection. The first is that you'll need to embrace change to decode your diagnosis and the second is to continuously seek positive outcomes for what is typically a difficult situation, as in, dealing with a chronic condition.

Progress is important, but joy is essential. If you don't learn to appreciate the journey, you'll always feel like you're running toward something just out of reach.

Finding Joy In The Journey

Now, celebrating progress, no matter how small, creates momentum and allows you to discover how these moments strengthen your alignment across Mind, Body, and Soul and inspire you to continue on your Pathway with confidence.

Momentum is the unsung hero of transformation. While grand achievements like sending prostate disease and cancer into remission make for great headlines, it's the small consistent victories that pave the way for real progress.

Why Celebrating Wins Matters

Think back to the last time you accomplished something meaningful. Maybe it was small, like taking a walk on a tough day, or big, like hitting a long-term health goal. How did it feel? For most Titans, these moments carry a spark of hope as a reminder that progress is possible, even in the face of challenges.

Celebrating wins is more than just an act of acknowledgment; it's a way to honor the journey. Each celebration strengthens:

- **Your Mind:** By focusing on progress, you create positive neural pathways that encourage resilience and optimism.
- **Your Body:** Physical celebrations, whether it's a fist pump or a moment of rest, energize you and remind you to honor your efforts.

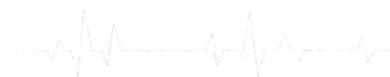

- **Your Soul:** Recognizing your achievements reconnects you with purpose and joy, reminding you that you are capable of incredible things.

Turning Progress Into a Habit

One of the most powerful ways to sustain motivation is to create rituals around celebrating wins. These rituals don't have to be extravagant. In fact, the simpler, the better. Here's how you can bring celebration into your daily life:

- **Start acknowledging wins:** Each day, write down one thing you did well. It might be as simple as drinking an extra glass of water or getting outside for five minutes. Over time, you'll have a collection of wins to look back on as a testament to your strength and perseverance.
- **Create Personal Rituals:** Light a candle, treat yourself to a favorite book, or take a deep breath and smile. Small gestures can make a big impact.
- **Share Your Wins:** Tell a trusted friend or community member. Saying your wins out loud reinforces their significance and creates a sense of shared joy.

Reflecting on Your Progress

Let's pause for a moment. What's one thing you've done today that makes you proud? Maybe it's showing up to read this chapter, or perhaps it's a choice you made to care for yourself. Whatever it is, take a moment to acknowledge it. These small reflections are the seeds of resilience, and with each one, you're building a stronger foundation for the journey ahead.

When you reflect on your progress, you're not just celebrating, you're setting the stage for future success. Think of it as watering a garden. Every acknowledgment of progress is a drop of water that helps your confidence and strength grow.

The Momentum of Joy

Celebrating progress is more than just a practice, it's a mindset. By shifting your focus to wins, no matter how small, you're creating momentum that carries you through the challenges. Each victory, whether it's a giant leap or a tiny step, is proof of your resilience and growth. The journey is about more than reaching the destination. It's about finding joy in every step along the way.

Take a deep breath. Smile. You've come so far already, and there's so much more waiting for you. In the next chapter, we'll explore how to navigate setbacks with resilience, turning challenges into opportunities for even greater growth.

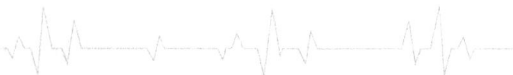

In the next chapter we'll take a look at the reality that along the way there are setbacks and how not to ignore them by navigating with resilience.

Fama's Sidebar: Recognizing Your Progress

Every step forward is worth celebrating. Remember, progress isn't always about big leaps, sometimes it's the small, steady steps that make the biggest difference. Take a moment today to reflect on how far you've come. What's one win you can celebrate right now? You're doing amazing, and I'm here cheering you on.

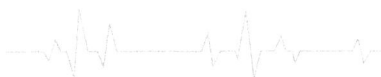

CHAPTER 23

Welcome to
The Titans Arena

For many, a diagnosis brings a profound sense of isolation, like standing in a crowded room yet feeling utterly alone. Studies reveal that individuals who engage with supportive communities often experience better emotional well-being and resilience, underscoring the transformative power of connection. The weight of your journey, the uncertainty of what lies ahead, and the lack of a shared space to connect with others who truly understand can make the process feel insurmountable. But what if you didn't have to face it alone? What if there was a place designed specifically for Titans like you, a dedicated, private, and safe community where you could find encouragement, wisdom, and connection?

This is the vision of *The Titans Arena*.

The Titans Arena is more than a community; it is a lifeline, a sanctuary, and a source of collective strength. Picture a space where you can share your journey without judgment, receive wisdom from those who have walked a similar path, and find encouragement to take the next step forward, this is the heart of the Arena. Built on the principles of decoding philosophy, the Arena fosters an environment where your Mind, Body, and Soul can find alignment through connection with others on similar paths. Here, you will discover a network of Titans who understand your challenges, celebrate your wins, and walk alongside you as you navigate your journey.

Why Community Matters

One of the greatest struggles Titans face is the sense of going it alone. It's natural to want to keep your burdens to yourself, especially when vulnerability feels risky or when support networks fall short of understanding the nuances of your experience. Yet, as studies and lived experiences show, community is a powerful antidote to isolation. It amplifies resilience, strengthens emotional wellbeing, and provides the shared wisdom that only peers can offer.

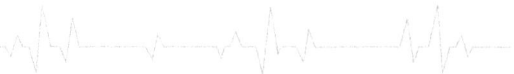

The concept of The Titans Arena arose from a personal need. While my support team was empathetic and supportive, at times I felt isolated. No one close to me truly understood what it meant to experience the condition first-hand.

There were times I longed to compare notes with someone who had walked this path before me. I first experienced a true Titanic bond with a close friend of my cousin. We were attending a wedding when I struck up a conversation with his friend, who had been through prostate cancer years earlier. He candidly shared his experiences recovering from incontinence and regaining sexual function. That conversation gave me a profound sense of reassurance. Finally, I had spoken with someone who understood. His honesty provided insights and encouragement that no textbook or medical professional could offer.

Without peers who truly comprehend their journey, the path forward can feel lonely and daunting.

Without community, challenges often feel heavier, and progress may come more slowly.

Finding someone with the same diagnosis can be challenging, especially for rare or severe conditions. Sometimes, they appear in unexpected places like my local yoga group. There, I met a fellow yogi with a similar vascular condition.

While our approaches to managing the condition were different, our discussions were invaluable. He had learned techniques that I hadn't considered, and I had insights that were new to him. We exchanged notes on what had worked, what hadn't, and how to approach daily challenges. We didn't expect to find solutions in every conversation, but the reassurance of knowing someone else understood made all the difference.

This type of connection reminds me why The Titans Arena is so vital. It creates a space where Titans can come together, share wisdom, and learn from one another's lived experiences.

Without the understanding of others who have faced similar challenges, every small victory feels muted, and setbacks feel insurmountable. But with the right connections, you gain not only support but also tools and insight to thrive.

Enter The Titans Arena

Imagine stepping into a space where everyone understands. Where your story matters and is met with empathy, not judgment. This is The Titans Arena, a dedicated online network designed for Titans who are ready to share, grow, and support one another.

In The Titans Arena, you'll find privacy and respect are at the core of this community. You can share your experiences knowing you're surrounded by others who get it.

Shared Wisdom

Access to practical advice, personal stories, and the collective insights of Titans who have faced similar challenges.

Encouragement and Empowerment

Whether you're celebrating a small win or navigating a setback, the Arena is here to cheer you on and lift you up.

This is more than a community; it's an extension of your own efforts, offering support and alignment for your Mind, Body, and Soul.

Success: The Transformation

By joining The Titans Arena, you're stepping into a space that will support you in your journey.

Judgment-free connections empower Titans to navigate their condition with confidence. Unlike casual conversations with friends or family who, despite their best intentions, may not fully grasp the experience. Instead, discussions within a community of Titans feel safer.

I've found that I can talk more openly with another Titan about fears surrounding my prognosis or even the possibility of death.

I was recently talking with a fellow Titan I'll call Tom, and the topic of cancer came up. In his case he had been in remission for two years after being diagnosed with Lymphoma. Now let's reflect on his severity for a minute. In my case, prostate cancer itself was not the concern, secondary cancers like bone cancer and lymphoma were. So on the scale of things Tom had received a crappy diagnosis and from the MRI shots he showed me it was the worst case I had seen. Tom's comments to me, about his relationship with his network, was what stood out. As a Titan with cancer "You can't be dark" about it or your team goes dark and focuses on the negative outcome because if they go dark "you'll be dead because everybody will focus on the negative outcome not the positive recovery". That's the sort of fresh, candid conversations you'll find in the arena.

These conversations, difficult as they may be, help to ease anxiety and provide clarity. It's the kind of connection that cannot be replicated outside of a shared experience.

The Titans Arena fosters this kind of support as a judgment-free space where Titans can find their voices, build confidence, and not be alone on their journey.

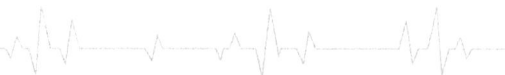

In your first few weeks, you might share your own experiences, receive actionable advice, and find encouragement that reignites your hope and determination. Imagine this:

You log in to the Arena and see a post from a fellow Titan who just reached a milestone you've been striving for. Their story inspires you, reminds you that progress is possible, and motivates you to keep going. You're not just a member of a community, you're part of a collective force of resilience and growth.

In the Arena, you'll find:

- **Strength in Numbers:** A network of Titans who share your challenges and triumphs.
- **Renewed Perspective:** Stories and insights that spark hope and inspire action.
- **Lasting Connections:** Relationships that transcend the challenges of today and provide ongoing support for tomorrow.

Call-to-Action

Join us in The Titans Arena today by visiting by clicking on this link to **register your interest.**

This is your invitation to a community where you'll find support, encouragement, and the shared strength of Titans just like you. Take the step, and let's walk this Pathway together.

In the final chapter, we'll celebrate the journey and look ahead to the boundless possibilities that await.

Fama's Sidebar

The Titans Arena is your space, a community of resilience and shared strength. What do you hope to gain from being part of a supportive community? Reflect on how connection can inspire growth and resilience. Take the first step by registering today. You'll find support, inspiration, and a network of Titans walking this journey with you.

CHAPTER 24

The Knife Edge of Time

Every Titan eventually finds themselves standing on what I call the Knife Edge of Time, that razor-thin present moment where past lessons and future hopes converge. Behind you lies the weight of diagnosis, the trials you've endured, and the resilience you've uncovered. Ahead of you stretches a horizon of uncertainty and possibility. But here, in the present, is where the real journey unfolds.

The Knife Edge is not about fear of falling; it is about clarity. This is where your decisions matter most. This is where the Alignment Codex becomes more than theory, it becomes your lived story. On this edge, you carry both the scars and the strength of your past, while reaching toward the promise of what comes next.

Where You've Come From

You've come a long way.

From the first shock of diagnosis through the pages of this book, you've walked step by step into a deeper understanding of yourself. You've discovered the Alignment Codex as the living record of your Mind, Body, and Soul. You've seen how resilience is built not in isolation, but through alignment, small steps, and the wisdom of lived experience.

This first book has been about finding clarity and reclaiming agency. You now carry the tools to begin decoding your diagnosis so you or someone close to you can take ownership of their health, their choices, and their future. But the journey doesn't stop here.

Where You Stand Now

Before moving forward, pause here. This is the *Knife Edge of Now*, the space where your Mind, Body, and Soul converge in real time to find some form of dynamic harmony. It's not a perfect balance but it's good enough to work for you.

- **Mind:**
    - What stories are you telling yourself today?
    - Are they filled with doubt, or are they rooted in resilience?

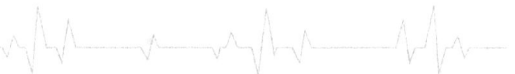

- **Body:**
  - How does your body feel right now?
  - Tired?
  - Strong?
  - Fragile?
  - Capable?
  - Every sensation is a signal, an invitation to listen more closely.

- **Soul:**
  - Where is your sense of meaning today?
  - Do you feel connected, inspired, or searching?
  - The Soul reminds us that even in struggle, there is purpose waiting to be claimed.

Take stock of yourself 'in this moment' now because this is where you live. This is not a test of perfection, it is a recognition that your present reality matters just as much as your past lessons or future goals.

Walking Forward Together

The road ahead isn't meant to be walked alone. That's why we created The Titans Arena as a dedicated community where Titans like us gather for encouragement, practical tools, and shared wisdom. Inside, you'll find not just connections, but real opportunities to keep moving forward.

- **The Alignment Campus** within The Arena hosts webinars, group coaching, and training programs designed to help you put these principles into practice.

- **Our Substack library** at *paulcobbin.com* offers a growing collection of resources: chapters, author's notes, behind-the-scenes chats, and ongoing reflections.

- **The ReadersKey™ subscription** on Substack takes you deeper, with weekly research-driven articles linked to the book's chapters, unpacking the science and reasoning behind Decode Your Diagnosis.

Your Next Step

Take a moment to celebrate how far you've come. You've done the hard work of starting. Now, keep that momentum alive. Step into The Arena. Explore the Campus programs. Dive into the ReadersKey library. Surround yourself with others on the same path.

Remember: your diagnosis, or the diagnosis of someone close to you, does not define you. How you respond to it does. The Alignment Codex you now carry is your foundation. The Arena is your community. The future is your legacy, and it is still yours to shape.

Welcome to the journey ahead.

Practical Reflections

Take a moment on the Knife Edge of Now. Write a short note to yourself capturing:

- **Mind:** One thought or belief you want to carry forward.
- **Body:** One action or habit that supports your well-being today.
- **Soul:** One source of meaning, joy, or connection you want to nurture.

Keep this note close, it's your compass for the next step of your journey.

Key Insight

The Knife Edge of Time reminds us that transformation doesn't happen in the abstract, it happens here, in the present. By honoring your past, recognizing your present, and stepping with intention toward the future, you move from being defined by a diagnosis to defining your own path as a Titan.

Fama's Sidebar: Your Navigator's Voice

Standing on the Knife Edge of Now can feel daunting, but it is also the most powerful place you can be. Every breath, every choice, every small step forward shapes your Codex and your future. Pause and ask yourself: What one action today brings my *Mind, Body, and Soul into better alignment?*

Remember, Titan, you don't have to walk this road alone. The Arena is waiting.

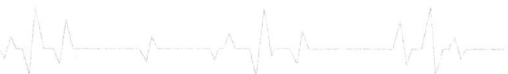

Unlock Action Now With The Alignment Workbook

Reading *Decode Your Diagnosis* is a powerful step but information alone doesn't change a life. What changes a life is action. And for Titans, whether you are living with a diagnosis, caring for someone you love, or supporting patients in a clinical role, action can feel overwhelming without the right tools.

That's why *The Alignment Workbook* exists. It's not another journal to collect dust on your nightstand. It's a structured, practical guide designed to help you apply the ideas you've just read. Inside, you'll find simple check-ins, clear exercises, and small alignment actions that give you momentum, clarity, and hope.

For the patient, this workbook helps you turn theory into daily progress. For the carer, it creates shared language and practices to walk alongside the one you love. And for the clinician, it offers a way to integrate the Decode Your Diagnosis framework into conversations and support beyond the clinic walls.

This is your action tool. A bridge from theory to practice. A way to move from simply *understanding* your diagnosis to actively *decoding it*, one step at a time.

Visit the Decode Your Diagnosis website to grab your copy now from:

decodeyourdiagnosis.com

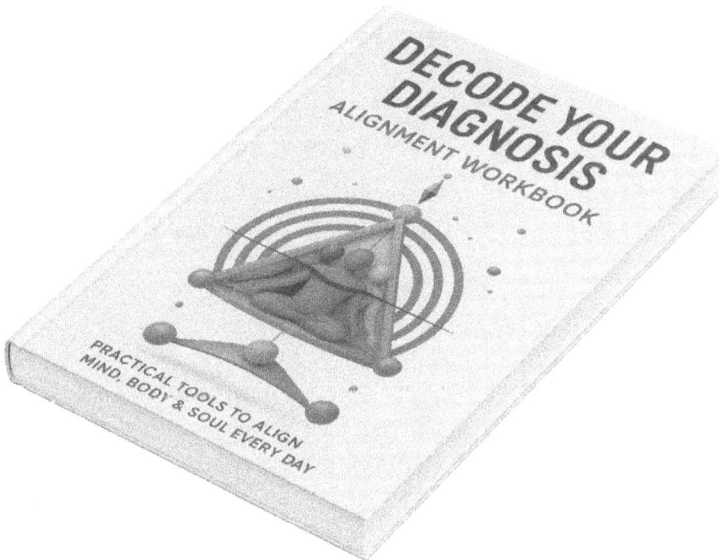

Epilogue

From Paul Cobbin

Dear Titan,

As the founder of the Decode Your Diagnosis philosophy and the lead author of this book, I want to offer you my final words.

If you've reached this point, you've taken the first step in understanding the foundational philosophy of Decode Your Diagnosis. I sincerely thank you for reading this book and hope it has empowered you with the possibility of decoding your diagnosis. At the very least, I hope it has opened your eyes to the potential of a functionally integrated approach in navigating chronic conditions, not just for yourself, but for those around you.

You've worked through this book and perhaps even dedicated time to the companion *Alignment Workbook*. Through these pages, I hope you have uncovered new perspectives, tools, and possibilities, opportunities to mold your own Alignment Pathway in ways you never imagined.

As patients, our chronic conditions should not define us. As Titans, we must find no boundaries.

Above all, I hope one core message has been embedded deep into your psyche:

Your health is yours.

It doesn't belong to your doctor.
It doesn't belong to your partner.
It doesn't belong to your insurance company.
It belongs to **YOU**.

I'll repeat that again: YOUR HEALTH IS YOURS.

You owe it to yourself to be resilient.
You owe it to your loved ones to fight for your well-being.
You owe it to your future self to walk the *Knife Edge of Time*, to live fully in the present while shaping what lies ahead.

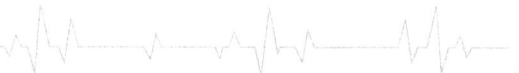

Decode Your Diagnosis provides the framework to be the most empowered Titan you've ever envisioned. Now, it's time to build your Pathway, step by step. Some steps will feel monumental. Others may feel like setbacks. But the Knife Edge of Now is in your favor, so make the most of it.

Feel free to use the tools in this book. They are no longer mine, they are yours. Adapt them, evolve them and discard what doesn't serve you. There is no perfect method, only the primary goal:

To Decode Your Diagnosis.

I've decoded my diagnosis a number of times. Now it's your turn.

Sincerely,

me@paulcobbin.com

Paul Cobbin

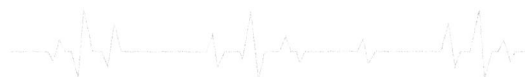

Appendix

Decoding Terms and Acronyms

This appendix provides definitions for the key terms and acronyms used throughout Decode Your Diagnosis. Understanding these concepts will help readers integrate the decoding Philosophy into their journey and apply the principles effectively.

Decoding Core Concepts

The Decode Your Diagnosis Philosophy

The foundational belief that Mind, Body, and Soul must work in harmony to achieve resilience, clarity, and well-being. This philosophy underpins all strategies in Decode Your Diagnosis.

The Three Elements

• **Mind** – The mental and emotional aspect of well-being, including thought patterns, decision-making, and cognitive resilience.

• **Body** – The physical component of health, including movement, nutrition, and medical interventions.

• **Soul** – The spiritual and purpose-driven aspect of life, including meaning, connection, and alignment with values.

Decoding Tools and Frameworks

The Alignment Codex

A structured representation of the *Decode Your Diagnosis* philosophy, serving as a philosophical foundation for *The Alignment Atlas*. The *Alignment Codex* encapsulates the values of courage, clarity, and resilience, guiding Titans toward alignment and long-term transformation.

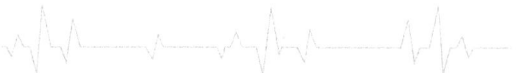

The Titans Arena

A dedicated supportive community where Titans connect, share experiences, and receive guidance from others who understand the challenges of a chronic diagnosis.

The Knife Edge of Time

A metaphor emphasizing that the present moment is the critical point where actions, choices, and alignment take place. The past provides lessons, the future offers possibilities, but transformation happens now.

Dynamic Harmony

The concept that balance is not static but an ongoing process of realignment across Mind, Body, and Soul as circumstances change.

Foundation Stone

The personalized compounding base for each Titan's journey, established by acknowledging their current state, setting realistic goals, and mapping a clear path forward.

Mindset and Psychological Strategies

Growth Mindset

A perspective that sees challenges as opportunities for learning and resilience, rather than obstacles or failures.

Empowered Diagnosis

A reframing of a medical diagnosis as an opportunity for personal growth and transformation, rather than a limitation.

Self-Compassion Practice

A structured method of treating oneself with kindness, patience, and understanding during difficult moments.

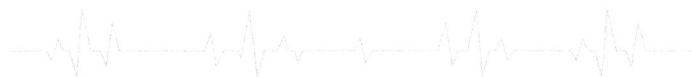

Reframing Limiting Beliefs

A technique for identifying and replacing negative thought patterns with more constructive and empowering perspectives.

Health and Wellness Terms

Functional Health Integration

A holistic approach that combines conventional medicine, functional medicine, Traditional Chinese Medicine (TCM), Ayurveda, and lifestyle interventions to optimize health outcomes.

Alignment Fitness

A comprehensive approach to physical, mental, and spiritual fitness that supports long-term health and well-being.

Heartfulness Meditation

A meditation technique that fosters deep emotional and mental alignment, used as a mindfulness practice in the decoding Philosophy.

AcuGraph Testing

A diagnostic tool used in Traditional Chinese Medicine (TCM) to measure meridian energy balance and identify areas needing intervention.

Meridian Energy Score

A measurement of overall wellness based on energy flow through the body's meridians, often used in acupuncture and holistic medicine.

Decoding Acronyms

CAD – Coronary Artery Disease

A condition that restricts blood flow to the heart due to plaque buildup in the arteries, also referred to in this book as "heart disease".

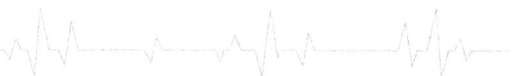

CSVD – Cerebral Small Vessel Disease

A condition affecting small blood vessels in the brain, leading to cognitive decline and increased stroke risk, also referred to in this book as "heart disease".

PCT – Porphyria Cutanea Tarda

A rare blood disorder that causes painful blisters and skin fragility in areas exposed to the sun. It's the most common type of porphyria.

T0 - Tzero

The moment of now, the only time where action is taking place and the moment that stays with, where you live life.

TCM – Traditional Chinese Medicine

A medical system incorporating herbal medicine, acupuncture, and meridian energy balance to support holistic healing.

Jing – Life Essence

A concept in Traditional Chinese Medicine that represents the body's core vitality, which can be preserved through balanced living and restorative practices.

This appendix serves as a quick reference guide for all Trinity-related terminology and concepts. By integrating these tools, Titans can confidently navigate their diagnosis and move toward a life of resilience, clarity, and empowerment.

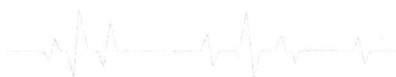

Unlock Action Now With The Alignment Workbook

Reading *Decode Your Diagnosis* is a powerful step but information alone doesn't change a life. What changes a life is action. And for Titans, whether you are living with a diagnosis, caring for someone you love, or supporting patients in a clinical role, action can feel overwhelming without the right tools.

That's why *The Alignment Workbook* exists. It's not another journal to collect dust on your nightstand. It's a structured, practical guide designed to help you apply the ideas you've just read. Inside, you'll find simple check-ins, clear exercises, and small alignment actions that give you momentum, clarity, and hope.

For the patient, this workbook helps you turn theory into daily progress. For the carer, it creates shared language and practices to walk alongside the one you love. And for the clinician, it offers a way to integrate the Decode Your Diagnosis framework into conversations and support beyond the clinic walls.

This is your action tool. A bridge from theory to practice. A way to move from simply *understanding* your diagnosis to actively *decoding* it, one step at a time.

Visit the Decode Your Diagnosis website to grab your copy now from:

decodeyourdiagnosis.com

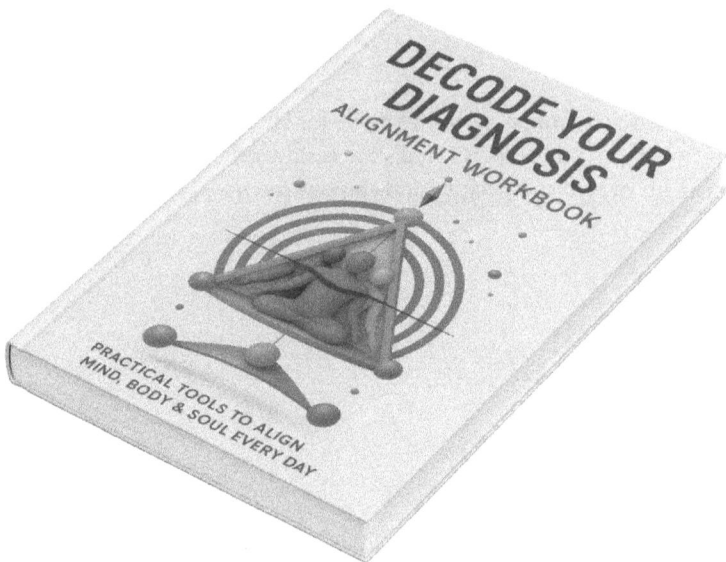

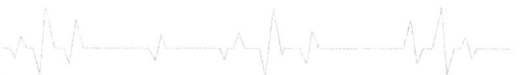

www.ingramcontent.com/pod-product-compliance
Lightning Source LLC
Chambersburg PA
CBHW031154020426
42333CB00013B/659